Endolumenal Therapy

Editor

STEVEN A. EDMUNDOWICZ

GASTROINTESTINAL ENDOSCOPY CLINICS OF NORTH AMERICA

www.giendo.theclinics.com

Consulting Editor
CHARLES J. LIGHTDALE

January 2013 • Volume 23 • Number 1

ELSEVIER

1600 John F. Kennedy Blvd. ● Suite 1800 ● Philadelphia, Pennsylvania 19103-2899

http://www.giendo.theclinics.com

GASTROINTESTINAL ENDOSCOPY CLINICS OF NORTH AMERICA Volume 23, Number 1
January 2013 ISSN 1052-5157, ISBN-13: 978-1-4557-7092-2

Editor: Kerry Holland
Developmental Editor: Donald Mumford

Gastrointestinal Endoscopy Clinics of North America (ISSN 1052-5157) is published quarterly by Elsevier Inc., 360 Park Avenue South, New York, NY 10010-1710. Months of issue are January, April, July, and October. Business and Editorial Offices: 1600 John F. Kennedy Blvd., Suite 1800, Philadelphia, PA, 19103-2899. Periodicals postage paid at New York, NY and additional mailing offices. Subscription prices are $315.00 per year for US individuals, $441.00 per year for US institutions, $168.00 per year for US students and residents, $351.00 per year for Canadian individuals, $538.00 per year for Canadian institutions, $445.00 per year for international individuals, $538.00 per year for international institutions, and $234.00 per year for Canadian and foreign students/residents. To receive student/resident rate, orders must be accompanied by name of affiliated institution, date of term, and the *signature* of program/residency coordinator on institution letterhead. Orders will be billed at individual rate until proof of status is received. Foreign air speed delivery is included in all *Clinics* subscription prices. All prices are subject to change without notice. **POSTMASTER:** Send address change to *Gastrointestinal Endoscopy Clinics of North America*, Elsevier Health Sciences Division, Subscription Customer Service, 3251 Riverport Lane, Maryland Heights, MO 63043. **Customer Service: 1-800-654-2452 (US). From outside the United States, call 1-314-447-8871. Fax: 1-314-447-8029. E-mail: JournalsCustomerService-usa@elsevier.com (for print support) or JournalsOnlineSupport-usa@elsevier.com (for online support).**

Reprints. For copies of 100 or more, of articles in this publication, please contact the Commercial Reprints Department, Elsevier Inc., 360 Park Avenue South, New York, NY 10010-1710. Tel. (212) 633-3812; Fax: (212) 482-1935; E-mail: reprints@elsevier.com.

Gastrointestinal Endoscopy Clinics of North America is covered in *Excerpta Medica, MEDLINE/PubMed (Index Medicus), and MEDLINE/MEDLARS.*

Printed and bound by CPI Group (UK) Ltd, Croydon, CR0 4YY

Transferred to digital print 2012

Contributors

CONSULTING EDITOR

CHARLES J. LIGHTDALE, MD
Professor, Department of Medicine, Columbia University Medical Center, New York, New York

GUEST EDITOR

STEVEN A. EDMUNDOWICZ, MD
Professor of Medicine, Chief of Endoscopy, Washington University School of Medicine, St Louis, Missouri

AUTHORS

A. AZIZ AADAM, MD
Instructor in Medicine-Gastroenterology and Hepatology, Northwestern University, Evanston, Illinois

GREGORY A. COTÉ, MD, MS
Assistant Professor of Medicine, Division of Gastroenterology and Hepatology, Department of Medicine, Indiana University School of Medicine, Indianapolis, Indiana

IHAB I. EL HAJJ, MD, MPH
Fellow, Division of Gastroenterology and Hepatology, Department of Medicine, Indiana University School of Medicine, Indianapolis, Indiana

BRINTHA K. ENESTVEDT, MD, MBA
Assistant Professor, Division of Gastroenterology, Temple University, Philadelphia, Pennsylvania

DAVID FRIEDEL, MD
Division of Gastroenterology, Hepatology and Nutrition, Department of Medicine, Winthrop University Hospital, Mineola; Adjunct Professor of Clinical Medicine, SUNY Stonybrook University School of Medicine, Stony Brook, New York

NORIO FUKAMI, MD, FASGE
Associate Professor of Medicine, Co-Director of Endoscopy, Director of Endoscopic Ultrasound, Division of Gastroenterology and Hepatology, University of Colorado Denver Anschutz Medical Campus, Aurora, Colorado

SRINIVAS GADDAM, MD, MPH
Division of Gastroenterology and Hepatology, Washington University School of Medicine, St Louis, Missouri

GREGORY G. GINSBERG, MD
Professor, Division of Gastroenterology, University of Pennsylvania, Philadelphia, Pennsylvania

TONYA KALTENBACH, MD, MS
Clinical Assistant Professor of Medicine (Affiliated), Veterans Affairs Palo Alto, Stanford University, Palo Alto, California

NITIN KUMAR, MD
Fellow, Division of Gastroenterology, Brigham and Women's Hospital, Boston, Massachusetts

STEVEN LEEDS, MD
Minimally Invasive Surgery Fellow, Providence Portland Medical Center, Portland, Oregon

JOHN A. MARTIN, MD
Associate Professor in Medicine-Gastroenterology and Hepatology and Surgery-Organ Transplantation, Director of Endoscopy, Northwestern University, Evanston, Illinois

RANI MODAYIL, MD
Division of Gastroenterology, Hepatology and Nutrition, Winthrop University Hospital, Mineola, New York

RAHUL PANNALA, MD
Division of Gastroenterology and Hepatology, Mayo Clinic, Scottsdale, Arizona

KEVIN REAVIS, MD, FACS
Esophageal and Foregut Surgery, Division of Gastrointestinal and Minimally Invasive Surgery, The Oregon Clinic, Portland, Oregon

ANDREW S. ROSS, MD
Digestive Disease Institute, Virginia Mason Medical Center, Seattle, Washington

ROY SOETIKNO, MD
Clinical Professor of Medicine (Affiliated), Veterans Affairs Palo Alto, Stanford University, Palo Alto, California

STAVROS N. STAVROPOULOS, MD
Division of Gastroenterology, Hepatology and Nutrition, Department of Medicine, Winthrop University Hospital, Mineola; Adjunct Professor of Clinical Medicine, College of Physicians and Surgeons, Columbia University, New York, New York

SHELBY SULLIVAN, MD
Assistant Professor of Medicine, Division of Gastroenterology, Center for Human Nutrition, Washington University School of Medicine, St Louis, Missouri

WATARU TAMURA, MD
Assistant Professor of Medicine, Division of Gastroenterology and Hepatology, University of Colorado Denver Anschutz Medical Campus, Aurora, Colorado

CHRISTOPHER C. THOMPSON, MD, MSc, FACG, FASGE
Director of Therapeutic Endoscopy, Brigham and Women's Hospital, Boston, Massachusetts

SACHIN WANI, MD
Division of Gastroenterology and Hepatology, Veterans Affairs Medical Center, University of Colorado, Denver; Assistant Professor of Medicine, Division of Gastroenterology and Hepatology, University of Colorado Anschutz Medical Campus, Aurora, Colorado

Contents

Foreword   **xi**

Charles J. Lightdale

Preface: Endolumenal Therapy of Gastrointestinal Disorders   **xiii**

Steven A. Edmundowicz

Endoscopic Therapy of Barrett Esophagus   **1**

Srinivas Gaddam and Sachin Wani

> Barrett esophagus (BE) is a well-established premalignant condition for esophageal adenocarcinoma (EAC), a lethal cancer with a dismal survival rate. The current guidelines recommend surveillance of patients with BE to detect dysplasia or early cancer before the development of invasive EAC. Recently, endoscopic eradication therapies have been shown to be safe and effective in the treatment of BE-related high-grade dysplasia and early EAC. This article reviews the various treatment options for BE and discusses the current evidence and gaps in knowledge in the understanding of treatment of this condition. In addition, recommendations are provided in context to the recently published guidelines by the American Gastroenterological Association.

Advances in Endoluminal Therapy for Esophageal Cancer   **17**

Brintha K. Enestvedt and Gregory G. Ginsberg

> Advances in endoscopic therapy have resulted in dramatic changes in the way early esophageal cancer is managed as well as in the palliation of dysphagia related to advanced esophageal cancer. Endoscopic mucosal resection (EMR) and endoscopic submucosal dissection (ESD) are effective therapies for accurate histopathologic staging and provide a potential for complete cure. Mucosal ablative techniques (radiofrequency ablation and cryotherapy) are effective adjuncts to EMR and ESD and reduce the occurrence of synchronous and metachronous lesions within the Barrett esophagus. The successes of these techniques have made endoscopic therapy the primary means of management of early esophageal cancer.

Endolumenal Therapies for Gastroesophageal Reflux Disease   **41**

Steven Leeds and Kevin Reavis

> TIF Stretta and Endocinch all seem technically safe in well-selected patients including those with prior esophageal and gastric surgeries. Long-term effectiveness is being evaluated. Given the current enthusiasm for increasingly less invasive surgical techniques, the inertia for endolumenal therapies continues to grow. Other endolumenal therapies for Gastroesophageal reflux disease (GERD) have initiated trials. These pursue similar fundoplication or lower esophageal sphincter reconstruction using simpler techniques with fewer steps. Because all endolumenal approaches

to GERD evolve, objective evaluation for symptom resolution and reduced esophageal acid exposure with improved esophagogastric physiology will remain a constant.

Achalasia   53

Stavros N. Stavropoulos, Rani Modayil, and David Friedel

Endoscopic therapy for achalasia is centered on disrupting or weakening the lower esophageal sphincter. The three traditional treatment options for achalasia are surgical myotomy, pneumatic dilation, and botulinum toxin injection. Pneumatic dilation yields results that are generally better than botulinum toxin injection and may approach a clinical response comparable with surgery. Per oral endoscopic myotomy is a newer endoscopic modality that will likely change the treatment paradigm for achalasia.

Early Gastric Cancer and Dysplasia   77

Wataru Tamura and Norio Fukami

Since the concept of early gastric cancer was first described in Japan in 1962, its treatment has evolved from curative surgical resection to endoscopic resection, initially with polypectomy to more recently with endoscopic submucosal dissection. As worldwide experience with these endoscopic techniques evolve and gain acceptance, studies have confirmed its comparable effectiveness with historical surgical outcomes in carefully selected patients. The criteria for endoscopic resection have expanded to offer more patients improved quality of life, avoiding the morbidity and mortality associated with surgery. This article summarizes the evolutional role of endoscopic and surgical therapy in early gastric cancer.

Endoscopic Diagnosis and Management of Ampullary Lesions   95

Ihab I. El Hajj and Gregory A. Coté

Most (>95%) ampullary lesions are adenomas or adenocarcinomas. Side viewing endoscopy, endoscopic ultrasound, and endoscopic retrograde cholangiopancreatography are complementary procedures that have an important role in the diagnosis, staging, and treatment of ampullary lesions. Here the authors review their epidemiology and discuss the evidence for endoscopic modalities, with an emphasis on techniques for endoscopic resection. Although endoscopic papillectomy represents one of the highest-risk endoscopic interventions, it has largely replaced surgical modalities for the treatment of adenomatous lesions. Appropriate patient selection and use of preventive maneuvers will minimize the likelihood of persistent or recurrent lesions and postprocedure complications.

Small Bowel Polyps, Arteriovenous Malformations, Strictures, and Miscellaneous Lesions   111

Rahul Pannala and Andrew S. Ross

Deep endoscopic access using double- and single-balloon enteroscopes and rotational endoscopy has vastly improved endoscopic therapeutic options in the small intestine. In this new era of interventional enteroscopy, significant advances have been made in the endoscopic treatment of small bowel polyps, angioectasias, and strictures. Although a decade ago small bowel polyps arising in the setting of a polyposis syndrome such as Peutz-Jeghers would have necessitated surgical resection, today endoscopic resection can typically be performed with positive clinical results. This article describes the current endoscopic management of small bowel polyps, arteriovenous malformations, strictures, and miscellaneous lesions identified within the small intestine.

Endoscopic Therapy for Postoperative Leaks and Fistulae   123

Nitin Kumar and Christopher C. Thompson

Endoscopic techniques for the treatment of postoperative fistulae and leaks are rapidly developing. Conventional surgical therapy for postsurgical leaks and fistulae is associated with significant morbidity and mortality. Novel endoscopic therapies have demonstrated safety, despite the inherent challenges of intervention in this patient population, and are steadily building evidence for efficacy relative to surgical management. The article examines endoscopic therapy for leaks and fistulae after esophageal, gastric, bariatric, colonic, and pancreaticobiliary surgery.

Endoscopic Resection of Large Colon Polyps   137

Tonya Kaltenbach and Roy Soetikno

Endoscopic resection, including polypectomy, endoscopic mucosal resection, and endoscopic submucosal dissection, is the preferred treatment method of large colorectal polyps. Its safety and efficacy have been shown. Endoscopic removal techniques are important because they provide a resection specimen for precise histopathologic staging to further direct diagnosis, prognosis, and management decisions. Used according to its indications, it provides curative resection and obviates the higher morbidity, mortality, and cost associated with alternative surgical treatment.

Enteral Stents in Malignant Bowel Obstruction   153

A. Aziz Aadam and John A. Martin

Enteral stent placement offers potentially improved quality of life, faster relief of obstructive symptoms, and is a minimally invasive alternative to surgery in patients with malignant bowel obstruction. Patients with malignant gastroduodenal obstruction and poor performance status are the best candidates for stent placement. Colonic stent placement as a bridge to surgery may be best reserved for patients with high pre-operative morbidity and mortality. Colonic stent placement should be avoided in patients receiving bevacizumab due to the increased risk of colonic perforation.

Endoscopy in the Management of Obesity   165

Shelby Sullivan

Obesity affects more than one third of adults in the United States and is associated with increased morbidity, mortality, and health care costs compared with normal weight adults. Current therapies include medical management consisting of therapeutic lifestyle change and pharmacotherapy, which has limited effectiveness, and bariatric surgery, which is currently the most effective therapy, but is limited by complications, long-term weight regain, and limited access. Endoscopic therapies are currently under investigation to treat weight regain after bariatric surgery and as a primary treatment for obesity, addressing the current gap in the treatment of obesity.

Index   **177**

GASTROINTESTINAL ENDOSCOPY CLINICS OF NORTH AMERICA

FORTHCOMING ISSUES

April 2013
Endoscopic Approach to the Patient with Biliary Tract Disease
Jacques Van Dam, MD, PhD,
Guest Editor

July 2013
Advanced Imaging in Endoscopy
Sharmila Anandasabapathy, MD,
Guest Editor

October 2013
Pancreatic Diseases
Martin Freeman, MD, *Guest Editor*

RECENT ISSUES

October 2012
Celiac Disease
Peter H.R. Green, MD, and
Benjamin Lebwohl, MD, *Guest Editors*

July 2012
Therapeutic ERCP
Michel Kahaleh, MD, *Guest Editor*

April 2012
Interventional Endoscopic Ultrasound
Kenneth J. Chang, MD, *Guest Editor*

RELATED INTEREST

Surgical Clinics of North America, October 2012 (Vol. 92, No. 5)
Contemporary Management of Esophageal Malignancy
Chadrick E. Denlinger, MD, and Carolyn E. Reed, MD, *Guest Editors*

NOW AVAILABLE FOR YOUR iphone and iPad

Foreword

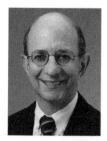

Charles J. Lightdale, MD
Consulting Editor

Gastroenterology, a subspecialty of Internal Medicine, started out with a heavy emphasis on contemplative diagnosis. Therapy was primarily with medications, and certainly the pharmacological treatment of gastrointestinal illness has grown exponentially. Gastrointestinal endoscopy also started as a diagnostic endeavor, and even the use of endoscopy-guided biopsy had a controversial start, only later becoming an essential element in endoscopic diagnosis. Therapeutic endoscopy was really jump-started with the development of the wire-snare electrocautery device for colonoscopic polypectomy. Since then, endoscopic therapies have multiplied to the point that some gastrointestinal endoscopists have created a new field of interventional endoscopy devoted primarily to invasive and therapeutic procedures.

Therapeutic endoscopic procedures have been applied via the mouth or rectum throughout the gastrointestinal tract. Many of these therapies can be applied by general gastroenterologists and are considered basic to endoscopic practice, while others require special training for organ-based specialists or interventionalists. I thought it might make a great issue of the *Gastrointestinal Endoscopy Clinics of North America* to cover the whole field of therapeutic endoscopy rather than focus on a specific technique or organ. It is extremely fortunate that Dr Steven Edmundowicz agreed to be the guest editor for this issue on the "Endolumenal Therapy of Gastrointestinal Disorders." By virtue of his skill and thoughtful, practical approach, Dr Edmundowicz has long been in the forefront of therapeutic endoscopy. He has chosen a wonderful group of author-experts to cover a broad array of topics. This "how-to-fix-it" issue of the *Gastrointestinal Endoscopy Clinics of North America* relates to every gastrointestinal endoscopist and is not to be missed.

Charles J. Lightdale, MD
Department of Medicine
Columbia University Medical Center
161 Fort Washington Avenue, Room 812
New York, NY 10032, USA

E-mail address:
CJL18@columbia.edu

Gastrointest Endoscopy Clin N Am 23 (2013) xi
http://dx.doi.org/10.1016/j.giec.2012.11.001
giendo.theclinics.com

Preface

Endolumenal Therapy of Gastrointestinal Disorders

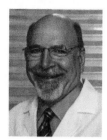

Steven A. Edmundowicz, MD
Guest Editor

We have witnessed amazing progress in the endoscopic therapy of gastrointestinal disorders over the past 2 decades. Endoscopic procedures that are now often completed in the outpatient setting have replaced what once were major operative interventions for our patients. This expansion of endolumenal therapies has transformed our approach to specific clinical problems in such a way that endoscopic therapy is now the preferred treatment option for many conditions discussed in this edition. This movement has offered exciting opportunities for endoscopists, biomedical engineers, and device developers while clearly benefitting our patients. It has also led to continued research and product development that promises to maintain and even accelerate progress in this arena in the coming years.

In this issue of *Gastrointestinal Endoscopy Clinics of North America* selected experts in specific clinical areas have described the significant progress that has occurred in endolumenal therapy of gastrointestinal disorders. Articles focus on specific issues from the esophagus to the colon and the applicable regions in between. Each article highlights the state-of-the-art approach to specific clinical disorders. Many individuals will enjoy reading the entire text for an overview of the direction the field of endolumenal therapy has taken. Others can alternatively focus only on specific articles of interest based on their practice or research field. Regardless, I am certain that you will find the articles well written and state of the art.

A work of this scope is not possible without the detailed contribution of the experts who have generously given their time and expertise to this project. For your contributions we are all sincerely grateful. A special thanks to Dr Charlie Lightdale for initiating this project and to Kerry Holland, the Senior Editor at Elsevier, for getting it all done. Please enjoy this issue of *Gastrointestinal Endoscopy Clinics of North America* on Endolumenal Therapy of Gastrointestinal Disorders. I hope it stimulates you to think about

Gastrointest Endoscopy Clin N Am 23 (2013) xiii–xiv
http://dx.doi.org/10.1016/j.giec.2012.10.012
1052-5157/13/$ – see front matter © 2013 Elsevier Inc. All rights reserved.

how you might modify your practice and improve patient care with even just one of these approaches.

Steven A. Edmundowicz, MD
Washington University School of Medicine
Campus Box 8124
660 S. Euclid Avenue
St Louis, MO 63110, USA

E-mail address:
SEdmundo@DOM.wustl.edu

Endoscopic Therapy of Barrett Esophagus

Srinivas Gaddam, MD, MPH[a], Sachin Wani, MD[b,c],*

KEYWORDS

- Barrett esophagus • Esophageal adenocarcinoma • Endoscopic therapy
- Dysplasia • Endoscopic mucosal resection • Radiofrequency ablation

KEY POINTS

- Accurate diagnosis and careful detailed inspection of the Barrett segment, using high-definition white light endoscopy, is an essential part of endoscopic evaluation of patients with Barrett esophagus (BE).
- The extent of BE should be defined using standardized reporting criteria, such as the Prague C & M classification, and all visible lesions in the Barrett segment should be described using the Paris classification.
- Endoscopic eradication therapy (EET) have been shown to be safe and effective in the treatment of Barrett-related neoplasia. Efficacy of radiofrequency ablation in the treatment of Barrett-related neoplasia has been demonstrated in a randomized controlled trial.
- The current AGA guidelines recommend against the requirement for use of chromoendoscopy, NBI, or any other advanced imaging for routine surveillance of patients with BE.
- According to the current AGA guidelines:
  - EET is only recommended to patients who develop HGD and intramucosal cancer.
  - In patients with confirmed LGD, the option to treat should be based on a shared decision between the patient and physician.
  - Surveillance is recommended for all patients with BE without dysplasia.

INTRODUCTION

Barrett esophagus (BE) is defined as the presence of metaplastic columnar-lined esophagus of any length on endoscopy and the presence of intestinal metaplasia on biopsy.[1] Approximately, 10% to 15% of patients with gastroesophageal reflux

---

Disclosure: No conflicts of interest relevant to this publication.
[a] Division of Gastroenterology and Hepatology, Washington University School of Medicine, 660 South Euclid Avenue, Campus Box 8124, St Louis, MO 63110-1093, USA; [b] Division of Gastroenterology and Hepatology, Veterans Affairs Medical Center, University of Colorado, 1055 Clermont Street, Denver, CO 80220, USA; [c] Division of Gastroenterology and Hepatology, University of Colorado Anschutz Medical Campus, 1635 Aurora Court, Room 2.031, Aurora, CO 80045, USA
* Corresponding author. Division of Gastroenterology and Hepatology, University of Colorado Anschutz Medical Campus, 1635 Aurora Court, Room 2.031, Aurora, CO 80045.
E-mail address: sachinwani10@yahoo.com

Gastrointest Endoscopy Clin N Am 23 (2013) 1–16
http://dx.doi.org/10.1016/j.giec.2012.10.001
giendo.theclinics.com

disease develop BE. BE is a well-established premalignant condition for esophageal adenocarcinoma (EAC),[1,2] a lethal cancer with a dismal survival rate (5-year survival of 15%). The incidence of EAC continues to increase at a greater rate (>500% increase since 1975)[3] than that of common cancers, such as breast, colon, lung, and prostate cancer.[4] Furthermore, in most patients, EAC has an insidious onset becoming clinically apparent only in advanced stages.

Patients with BE are generally thought to progress through stages of dysplasia (low-grade dysplasia [LGD] to high-grade dysplasia [HGD]), with progressive accumulation of abnormal genetic alterations, before finally progressing to EAC. To date, the only reliable predictor for EAC is the development of dysplasia and hence the current societal guidelines recommend surveillance of patients with BE to detect dysplasia or early cancer before the development of invasive EAC.[5–8]

For decades, patients developing HGD and mucosal cancer were traditionally treated with esophagectomy. Despite being the definitive therapy (by achieving resection of the precursor BE epithelium and the involved lymph nodes) esophagectomy carries a high risk of procedure-related long-term morbidity and mortality.[9,10] These unacceptably high rates of mortality and morbidity have fueled interest in other forms of less invasive therapy. During the last two decades, innovative endoscopic treatments have been shown to be safe and effective in the treatment of BE and early EAC. This has resulted in an array of endoscopic therapeutic options for patients with BE. This article reviews the various treatment options for BE and discusses the current evidence and gaps in knowledge in the understanding of treatment of this condition. In addition, recommendations are provided in context to the recently published guidelines by the American Gastroenterological Association (AGA).[11]

HISTOPATHOLOGY AND RATIONALE FOR ENDOSCOPIC ERADICATION THERAPY

There are worsening grades of cytologic and architectural changes on the continuum from LGD to invasive esophageal cancer. These are generally described as cytologic (stratified, hyperchromatic nuclei with nuclear enlargement, increased nuclear-to-cytoplasmic ratio, prominent nucleoli, increased mitotic figures, and loss of nuclear polarity) or architectural (crypt budding, branching, marked crowding, cribriform formation, and variation of crypt size and shape).[12,13] The current diagnoses of LGD, HGD, and EAC are based on the recommendations of the Vienna classification.[14] Intramucosal cancer is defined by the invasion of neoplasia into the surrounding lamina propria or muscularis mucosae but not into the submucosa. Presence of unequivocal stromal desmoplasia is consistent with submucosal EAC.[15,16]

Previously, patients with HGD and intramucosal cancer were routinely treated with esophagectomy.[17] Esophagectomy is considered to be a definitive therapy for BE because it resects the premalignant tissue along with the dysplastic lesion and the surrounding lymph nodes, and hence is considered to have very low risk of recurrence of cancer. In a retrospective study, cancer-free survival in 46 patients undergoing esophagectomy for T1a EAC in a tertiary care center was reported to be 95% at 5 years.[18] However, esophagectomy has been associated with a defined morbidity and mortality risk. This perception has led to the rapid development of endoscopic therapeutic options. Observational data suggest that endoscopic eradication therapy (EET) is highly effective and that the long-term survival in patients with HGD and early EAC is similar to those undergoing esophagectomy.[18–21] Moreover, a cost-effectiveness model of endoscopic ablation of HGD in patients with BE concluded that endoscopic ablation was more effective than surveillance or esophagectomy.[22] Previous surgical series have shown that in patients with HGD or intramucosal cancer, the risk of lymph node metastases is 0% to 3%.[23–27] A recent systematic review that included 1874 patients with HGD and mucosal EAC undergoing esophagectomy showed overall risk of lymph node metastasis of 1.39% (95% confidence interval [CI], 0.86–1.92). Specifically, in the group of patients with mucosal EAC the risk of lymph node metastases was 1.93% (95% CI, 1.19–2.66).[28] This compares favorably with the perioperative mortality rate associated with esophagectomy. In contrast, in patients with submucosal EAC, lymph node metastasis is reported in excess of 20% of cases.[25–27,29,30] Therefore, EET is recommended in patients with HGD or intramucosal cancer but not in patients with EAC involving the submucosa.[12]

ACCURATE DIAGNOSIS AND STAGING
Role of Advanced Imaging and Endoscopic Ultrasound

Careful and detailed examination with high-definition white light endoscopy of the Barrett segment is an essential part of the management of patients with BE. A recent study showed that inspecting the mucosa for more than 1 minute per cm length of Barrett segment was more likely to detect HGD/EAC,[31] underscoring the importance of detailed inspection of the Barrett mucosa. The extent of BE should be defined using standardized reporting criteria, such as the Prague C & M classification.[32] The morphology of visible lesions can have a bearing on the T-staging because nonprotruding, superficial lesions are likely to be associated with submucosal invasion.[33] Therefore, all visible lesions in the Barrett segment should be described using the Paris classification (**Fig. 1**).[33]

Significant strides have been made in advanced imaging techniques to identify early neoplasia in patients with BE. Advanced imaging technologies, such as narrow band imaging (NBI), autofluorescence imaging, confocal laser endomicroscopy (CLE), and optical coherence tomography, have a role in characterization of visible lesions and detection of flat dysplasia. High-definition endoscopy has been shown to have a higher sensitivity in the detection of Barrett-related neoplasia when compared with standard endoscopy and should be the present standard of care. NBI offers the benefits of

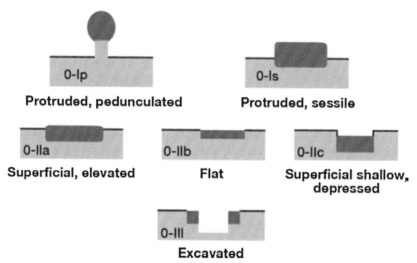

Fig. 1. A diagram illustrating the Paris classification. (*From* The Paris endoscopic classification of superficial neoplastic lesions: esophagus, stomach, and colon: November 30 to December 1, 2002. Gastrointest Endosc 2003;58:S3–43; with permission.)

chromoendoscopy while making it easy and simple by providing an on-demand, push-button technique to better characterize the mucosal and vascular patterns in detecting dysplasia. These patterns have a high sensitivity and specificity in the detection of dysplasia within the Barrett segment. In a multicenter, randomized, crossover trial of 123 patients, there was no significant difference in detection of dysplasia between routine four-quadrant white light endoscopy biopsies and NBI-directed biopsies; however, NBI required fewer biopsies (3.6 vs 7.6 biopsies per procedure; P = .001).[34] NBI and autofluorescence imaging are considered to be red flag or broad-field technologies that are used to identify dysplastic lesions. A relatively newer technology, CLE, enables real-time, in vivo evaluation of histology. A multicenter randomized controlled trial showed a significant improvement in detection of HGD/EAC with a probe-based CLE.[35] Recently, probe-based CLE criteria for the diagnosis of dysplasia were scientifically created, tested, and validated in BE.[36–38] These criteria were found to have a high degree of overall accuracy and interobserver variability. Although not ready for prime-time, these are exciting times for advanced imaging techniques and future studies should define its role in the management of patients with BE. The current AGA guidelines recommend against the use of chromoendoscopy, NBI, or any other advanced imaging for routine surveillance of patients with BE.

Although the role of endoscopic ultrasound has been established in the accurate T and N staging of invasive EAC, recent studies have shown only a modest accuracy in delineating T-staging in patients with HGD and intramucosal EAC.[39–43] Recently, results from a US multicenter cohort of patients with BE (N = 105) assessing the diagnostic accuracy of endoscopic ultrasound in establishing T-stage (depth of invasion) using endoscopic mucosal resection (EMR) as the gold standard showed that the overall accuracy of endoscopic ultrasound was 72% (95% CI, 63–81). Presence or absence of visible lesions did not make a differences in the accuracy rates (69% vs 84%; P = .26).[44] Young and colleagues[39] reported a T-stage concordance rate of 65% in a systematic review, using EMR/surgical pathology as the gold standard. Based on these data, endoscopic ultrasound has a limited role in the evaluation of patients with early neoplasia.

Diagnostic Endoscopic Mucosal Resection

This technique involves the use of a diathermic snare or an endoscopic needle for resection of a neoplastic lesion or intestinal metaplasia to the level of submucosa. Accurate T-staging is critical in making therapeutic decisions in patients with dysplastic BE. EMR has evolved into an important diagnostic and therapeutic tool in the evaluation and management of BE-related neoplasia (**Fig. 2**). In a study comparing preoperative EMR with histologic examination on esophagectomy specimens, there was perfect agreement between the two.[45] Studies comparing routine biopsies of visible lesions with EMR report a 30% to 48% rate in change in diagnosis after obtaining an EMR.[46–48] Moreover, in a study comparing 251 EMR specimens with biopsy, EMR improved interobserver agreement among expert gastrointestinal pathologists when compared with biopsy specimens (κ = 0.43 vs 0.35 for HGD; P = .018).[49] This improvement in interobserver variability has been attributed to a larger tissue sample with limited architectural distortion. Although EMR is routinely recommended for visible lesions, the data are limited on its role in flat dysplasia.

ENDOSCOPIC ERADICATION THERAPIES AND SUPPORTING EVIDENCE

The primary goal of endoscopic therapy is to prevent the development of invasive EAC by treating the dysplastic lesion, thereby improving patient survival. However, patients

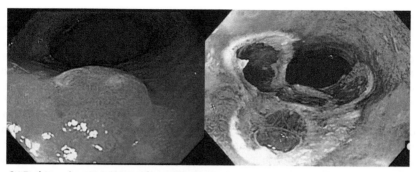

Fig. 2. Endoscopic appearance of a visible lesion in the Barrett's segment before and after EMR.

who develop dysplasia are at higher risk of recurrence of neoplasia and metachronous lesions from the remaining segment of BE, which occurs in up to 30% of patients undergoing EET.[50] Therefore, complete ablation of the entire Barrett segment should be the goal in all patients undergoing EET.

Radiofrequency Ablation

Radiofrequency ablation (RFA) uses a catheter with an inflatable balloon at its tip that is connected to an energy generator. This catheter is passed through the working channel of an endoscope. The balloon at the tip of the catheter has bipolar heating elements that can cause superficial tissue injury. When the balloon is inflated and radiofrequency energy is applied over a circumferential Barrett segment, it causes ablation of the mucosa that is in contact with the balloon and can treat 3 cm of circumferential BE with each application (**Fig. 3**). To treat smaller areas, such as islands, noncircumferential BE, and residual BE after treatment, a focal ablation device that works on the same principles of RFA is available. There is level 1 evidence demonstrating high rates of complete eradication of dysplasia and intestinal metaplasia in patients with BE with HGD and LGD.[51,52] In a randomized sham-controlled trial of 127 patients in an intention-to-treat analysis, complete eradication was achieved in 81% of patients with HGD who underwent RFA compared with 19% of control subjects ($P<.001$).[51] In

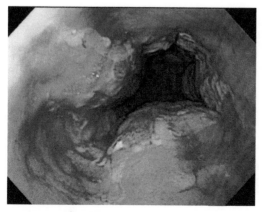

Fig. 3. Endoscopic appearance after RFA.

a follow-up cross-over of this study describing durability of RFA, after 3 years dysplasia remained eradicated in more than 85%, whereas intestinal metaplasia remained eradicated in more than 75% of patients without maintenance RFA.[53] Among 64 patients with LGD (42 RFA, 22 sham) included in this study,[51] at 1-year follow-up complete eradication rates of LGD (90% vs 23%; P<.001) and intestinal metaplasia (81% vs 4%; P<.001) were significantly higher in patients undergoing RFA when compared with control subjects. There is no randomized controlled trial demonstrating efficacy of RFA in patients with nondysplastic BE. In a multicenter study, patients with nondysplastic BE who had complete response to RFA 2.5 years after ablation were enrolled in a 5-year outcomes study.[54] Using per protocol analysis, they report a complete response to metaplasia in 92%. Based on Kaplan-Meier analysis, it is estimated that 91% of patients would have complete response and that the mean duration of complete response would be 4.2 years. The main strengths of this technique include a precise and controlled delivery of a predetermined standardized radiofrequency energy, simplicity and ease of procedure, and its association with low stricture rate.

Cryotherapy

Cryotherapy is a noncontact technique that involves tissue destruction of metaplastic epithelium by intracellular disruption and ischemia that is produced by "freeze-thaw" cycles using liquid nitrogen or carbon dioxide. This is delivered through a catheter that can be passed through the working channel of any endoscope. The targeted spray is directed toward the BE segment to effectively induce a freeze cycle. An orogastric tube is introduced to help removal of excessive nitrogen or carbon dioxide and hence prevent perforation of viscus. Multiple freeze and thaw cycles are induced in each segment of the Barrett epithelium to produce effective ablation (**Fig. 4**). The freeze-thaw cycles tend to cause intracellular damage while preserving the extracellular matrix and theoretically are thought to produce minimal fibrosis and effectively fewer strictures. Recent data suggest that cryotherapy is safe and effective in the treatment of HGD.[55–59] In a multicenter prospective study of 77 patients, complete response to cryotherapy was seen in 94% in patients with HGD (17 patients) and 100% in patients with EAC (7 patients).[58] In a retrospective study of 98 patients, complete eradication of HGD was seen in 97% of patients.[57] There are no randomized controlled trials evaluating the role of cryotherapy in BE-related neoplasia. Anecdotally, the use of

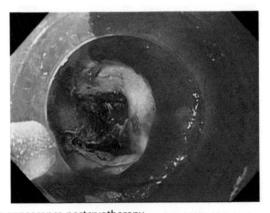

Fig. 4. Endoscopic appearance postcryotherapy.

cryotherapy is limited to patients who have developed post-EMR stricture and those who have failed to achieve complete remission with RFA.[12]

Endoscopic Resection of All BE

Endoscopic eradication using EMR alone involves focal EMR of visible lesions followed by complete eradication of the remaining Barrett segment with stepwise EMR.[46] Most experts believe that EMR resection of the entire Barrett segment can be performed in patients with Barrett segment length of less than or equal to 5 cm. There are several techniques of EMR, including cap-assisted EMR after saline lift and band ligation with snare resection (multiband mucosectomy). A randomized controlled trial comparing these two techniques demonstrated that there is no difference in the thickness of specimen and resection of submucosa; however, the multiband ligation technique had a shorter procedure time and produced smaller EMR specimens.[60] Based on several case series, the complete eradication of neoplasia and intestinal metaplasia ranges from 85.4% to 100% and 75.6% to 97%, respectively.[46,47,61–63] In a study with 169 patients, after a median follow-up of 32 months, the eradication of neoplasia and intestinal metaplasia was found to be durable (95.3% and 80.5%, respectively).[62] In this technique, despite EMR being the primary tool for treatment of dysplasia and intestinal metaplasia, touch-up treatments with argon plasma coagulation may be required. One of the strengths of stepwise EMR as a modality for complete resection of the Barrett segment includes the availability of tissue for histologic evaluation. However, there are significant risks that have been reported: bleeding in 0% to 46%,[18,46,63–66] perforation in 1% to 5%,[63,67] and strictures in 2% to 88% of patients undergoing complete EMR of the Barrett segment.[61–63,68–71]

Multimodal EET

Multimodality EET involves the initial performance of EMR of visible lesions or abnormal mucosal patterns on advanced imaging followed by eradication of intestinal metaplasia in the remaining Barrett segment by using mucosal ablative techniques, such as RFA, cryotherapy, or argon plasma coagulation.

A multicenter prospective study of 24 patients found RFA after initial diagnostic EMR of visible lesions to be safe and effective.[72] A retrospective analysis comparing histologic outcomes and complication rates between patients that underwent RFA therapy after an initial diagnostic EMR and those who underwent only RFA therapy showed comparable rates of dysplasia and strictures.[73] In a case series report of 349 patients that received multimodal therapy (EMR, photodynamic therapy, and argon plasma coagulation), complete eradication was achieved in 94.5% and a long-term complete response was seen in 94.4%.[50] Predictors of recurrence of intestinal metaplasia after multimodality therapies were long-segment BE, multifocal neoplasia, piecemeal resection, receiving no ablative therapy after initial complete response, and more than 10 months duration to achieve complete response. A randomized controlled study, only one of its kind, comparing stepwise EMR and initial diagnostic EMR followed by RFA in patients with BE segment length of less than or equal to 5 cm with HGD and early EAC showed no difference between the two groups for complete eradication of dysplasia (100% vs 96%) and intestinal metaplasia (92% vs 96%). However, patients who underwent stepwise EMR were more likely to develop strictures (88% vs 14%; $P<.001$) and require more therapeutic endoscopies (6 vs 3; $P<.001$). Based on these data, it is recommended that patients with HGD and early EAC undergo EMR of visible lesion followed by RFA to the remaining Barrett segment for complete eradication of intestinal metaplasia.

CANDIDATES FOR EET

Candidacy for EET is based on the presence and grade of dysplasia that determines the future risk for the development of EAC. Based on recent population study estimates, the risk of developing cancer in patients with BE is very low (0.12% per year).[74] Variable annual rates of progression to cancer have been reported in patients with LGD (range, 0.4%–13%). However, patients with HGD are at the highest risk for progression to EAC (6.6% per year).[4,74–76]

High-Grade Dysplasia or Intramucosal Cancer

Given the high rate of progression to EAC, current AGA guidelines recommend EET rather than surveillance in the management of patients with HGD. With the available high-quality evidence, RFA is the preferred mucosal ablative technique after initial EMR of the visible lesions in the treatment of HGD and intramucosal EAC (**Fig. 5**).[11]

Low-Grade Dysplasia

There are several gaps in recognizing and understanding the natural history of LGD in BE.[77] Variability in the rates of progression to EAC[78–83] has been attributed to small sample size, unclear distinction between incident and prevalent LGD, referral bias, and lack of central pathology review.[77] In addition, there is poor interobserver agreement even among community and expert gastrointestinal pathologists ($\kappa = 0.14$–0.32).[76,78,84] Furthermore, several attempts at risk stratification of LGD based on unifocal or multifocal, incident or prevalent, or proximal or distal have not yielded success.[77] Several studies evaluating the role of ablative therapy have classified LGD with either nondysplastic BE or in the group with HGD, making evaluation of the efficacy and durability of EET in LGD difficult. Given these issues with unclear natural history, poor interobserver agreement, unclear risk stratification, and lack of established benefit of eradication, routine EET of patients with LGD is not recommended. Current AGA guidelines support the use of RFA as an option for the treatment of confirmed (by two pathologists) LGD. However, this should be considered on a case-by-case basis with informed shared decision making between the physician and the patient.[11]

Nondysplastic BE

Several techniques have been evaluated in patients with nondysplastic BE.[51,52,85–94] To date, there are no randomized controlled trials evaluating the role of ablative therapies compared with surveillance alone in nondysplastic BE. A recent cost-effectiveness study evaluating the role of EET with RFA in patients with nondysplastic BE showed the associated costs are prohibitively expensive.[95] In addition, there is no clear evidence that surveillance can be stopped after ablation. The number needed to treat to prevent one cancer (assuming an absolute risk reduction of EAC of 0.3% per year with ablation of nondysplastic BE) is estimated to be 333 patients per year.[96] Furthermore, several critical questions regarding the efficacy, durability, and costs remain unanswered. It is unclear whether the risks of endoscopic therapy outweigh benefits of ablation to reduce the already low risk of EAC. Considering the lack of data and several other unanswered questions, the current AGA guidelines do not recommend EET in patients with nondysplastic BE.[11]

COMPLICATIONS AND ISSUES POST-EET

The three major complications include (1) bleeding, (2) perforation, and (3) esophageal strictures. Esophageal stricture rate has been described to occur in about 8% of

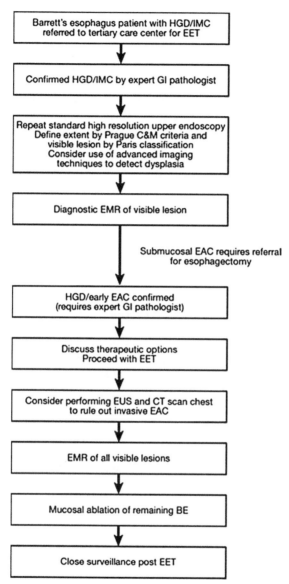

Fig. 5. Flow chart for the management of patients with BE with HGD and intramucosal EAC. (*From* Wani S, Early D, Edmundowicz S, et al. Management of high-grade dysplasia and intramucosal adenocarcinoma in Barrett's esophagus. Clin Gastroenterol Hepatol 2012;10(7): 704–11; with permission.)

patients treated with RFA, 9% to 14% of patients treated with multimodality EET, and 56% to 88% in patients undergoing stepwise EMR.[46,53,61,62] Overall, perforations have been described in less than 5% and bleeding in less than 10% of patients undergoing EET. Chest pain can occur in about 25% of patients undergoing EET. One of the other concerns of any EET is the development of subsquamous intestinal metaplasia, which continues to put the patient at risk for EAC.[97–104] The occurrence of subsquamous intestinal metaplasia poses a significant challenge to BE diagnosis because existing biopsy techniques do not adequately sample the lamina propria, as noted in a recent study demonstrating that only 37% of all biopsy specimens contained adequate lamina propria.[97] Variable sampling protocol, tangential sampling, and striping of biopsy specimens make it difficult to diagnose subsquamous intestinal metaplasia. A new technology, optical coherence tomography, offers promise in the detection of subsquamous intestinal metaplasia.[105–108] In addition, patients who have undergone complete eradication of BE are at risk for recurrence of intestinal metaplasia (about 25%) and dysplasia (about 10%–15% in patients undergoing RFA).[53] Unfortunately, because of these reasons, EET does not obviate the need for surveillance.

SUMMARY

Large epidemiologic studies show that the risk of EAC in patients with BE is very low; most patients with BE do not progress to cancer and die of other unrelated causes. However, the incidence of EAC has increased more than 500% in the last few decades. Given the availability of safe and effective endoscopic treatments, it is appealing to advocate EET of all patients with BE. This is, however, riddled with many problems including high costs, high burden of risks from treatment of large numbers of patients at low risk of EAC, and lack of long-term efficacy and durability data. To stem the rapid increase in EAC, it may be an effective strategy to endoscopically treat only those patients who are at high risk of progression to cancer. However, such risk stratification tools have so far been elusive. Until such a clinically useful tool is available, EET is only recommended to patients with HGD and intramucosal cancer. In patients with confirmed LGD the option to treat should be based on a shared decision between the patient and physician. Current guidelines recommend surveillance for patients with BE without dysplasia.

REFERENCES

1. Sharma P. Clinical practice. Barrett's esophagus. N Engl J Med 2009;361(26): 2548–56.
2. Lagergren J, Bergstrom R, Lindgren A, et al. Symptomatic gastroesophageal reflux as a risk factor for esophageal adenocarcinoma. N Engl J Med 1999; 340(11):825–31.
3. Pohl H, Welch HG. The role of overdiagnosis and reclassification in the marked increase of esophageal adenocarcinoma incidence. J Natl Cancer Inst 2005; 97(2):142–6.
4. Wani S, Falk G, Hall M, et al. Patients with nondysplastic Barrett's esophagus have low risks for developing dysplasia or esophageal adenocarcinoma. Clin Gastroenterol Hepatol 2011;9(3):220–7 [quiz: e26].
5. Wang KK, Sampliner RE, Practice Parameters Committee of the American College Gastroenterology. Updated guidelines 2008 for the diagnosis, surveillance and therapy of Barrett's esophagus. Am J Gastroenterol 2008;103(3): 788–97.
6. Spechler SJ, Sharma P, Souza RF, et al. American Gastroenterological Association technical review on the management of Barrett's esophagus. Gastroenterology 2011;140(3):e18–52 [quiz: e13].
7. Playford RJ. New British Society of Gastroenterology (BSG) guidelines for the diagnosis and management of Barrett's oesophagus. Gut 2006;55(4):442.

8. Boyer J, Laugier R, Chemali M, et al. French Society of Digestive Endoscopy SFED guideline: monitoring of patients with Barrett's esophagus. Endoscopy 2007;39(9):840–2.
9. van Lanschot JJ, Hulscher JB, Buskens CJ, et al. Hospital volume and hospital mortality for esophagectomy. Cancer 2001;91(8):1574–8.
10. Swisher SG, Deford L, Merriman KW, et al. Effect of operative volume on morbidity, mortality, and hospital use after esophagectomy for cancer. J Thorac Cardiovasc Surg 2000;119(6):1126–32.
11. American Gastroenterological Association, Spechler SJ, Sharma P, et al. American Gastroenterological Association medical position statement on the management of Barrett's esophagus. Gastroenterology 2011;140(3):1084–91.
12. Wani S, Early D, Edmundowicz S, et al. Management of high-grade dysplasia and intramucosal adenocarcinoma in Barrett's esophagus. Clin Gastroenterol Hepatol 2012;10(7):704–11.
13. Goldblum JR. Barrett's esophagus and Barrett's-related dysplasia. Mod Pathol 2003;16(4):316–24.
14. Schlemper RJ, Riddell RH, Kato Y, et al. The Vienna classification of gastrointestinal epithelial neoplasia. Gut 2000;47(2):251–5.
15. Odze RD. Diagnosis and grading of dysplasia in Barrett's oesophagus. J Clin Pathol 2006;59(10):1029–38.
16. Downs-Kelly E, Mendelin JE, Bennett AE, et al. Poor interobserver agreement in the distinction of high-grade dysplasia and adenocarcinoma in pretreatment Barrett's esophagus biopsies. Am J Gastroenterol 2008;103(9):2333–40 [quiz: 2341].
17. Spechler SJ. Dysplasia in Barrett's esophagus: limitations of current management strategies. Am J Gastroenterol 2005;100(4):927–35.
18. Prasad GA, Wu TT, Wigle DA, et al. Endoscopic and surgical treatment of mucosal (T1a) esophageal adenocarcinoma in Barrett's esophagus. Gastroenterology 2009;137(3):815–23.
19. Prasad GA, Wang KK, Buttar NS, et al. Long-term survival following endoscopic and surgical treatment of high-grade dysplasia in Barrett's esophagus. Gastroenterology 2007;132(4):1226–33.
20. Pech O, Bollschweiler E, Manner H, et al. Comparison between endoscopic and surgical resection of mucosal esophageal adenocarcinoma in Barrett's esophagus at two high-volume centers. Ann Surg 2011;254(1):67–72.
21. Das A, Singh V, Fleischer DE, et al. A comparison of endoscopic treatment and surgery in early esophageal cancer: an analysis of surveillance epidemiology and end results data. Am J Gastroenterol 2008;103(6):1340–5.
22. Inadomi JM, Somsouk M, Madanick RD, et al. A cost-utility analysis of ablative therapy for Barrett's esophagus. Gastroenterology 2009;136(7):2101–2114.e1–6.
23. Peyre CG, DeMeester SR, Rizzetto C, et al. Vagal-sparing esophagectomy: the ideal operation for intramucosal adenocarcinoma and Barrett with high-grade dysplasia. Ann Surg 2007;246(4):665–71 [discussion: 671–4].
24. Oh DS, Hagen JA, Chandrasoma PT, et al. Clinical biology and surgical therapy of intramucosal adenocarcinoma of the esophagus. J Am Coll Surg 2006;203(2): 152–61.
25. Stein HJ, Feith M, Bruecher BL, et al. Early esophageal cancer: pattern of lymphatic spread and prognostic factors for long-term survival after surgical resection. Ann Surg 2005;242(4):566–73 [discussion: 573–5].
26. Feith M, Stein HJ, Siewert JR. Pattern of lymphatic spread of Barrett's cancer. World J Surg 2003;27(9):1052–7.

27. Rice TW, Zuccaro G Jr, Adelstein DJ, et al. Esophageal carcinoma: depth of tumor invasion is predictive of regional lymph node status. Ann Thorac Surg 1998;65(3):787–92.

28. Dunbar KB, Spechler SJ. The risk of lymph-node metastases in patients with high-grade dysplasia or intramucosal carcinoma in Barrett's esophagus: a systematic review. Am J Gastroenterol 2012;107(6):850–62 [quiz: 863].

29. Konda VJ, Waxman I. Endotherapy for Barrett's esophagus. Am J Gastroenterol 2012;107:827–33.

30. Luna RA, Gilbert E, Hunter JG. High-grade dysplasia and intramucosal adeno-carcinoma in Barrett's esophagus: the role of esophagectomy in the era of endo-scopic eradication therapy. Curr Opin Gastroenterol 2012;28(4):362–9.

31. Gupta N, Gaddam S, Wani SB, et al. Longer inspection time is associated with increased detection of high-grade dysplasia and esophageal adenocarcinoma in Barrett's esophagus. Gastrointest Endosc 2012;76(3):531–8.

32. Sharma P, Dent J, Armstrong D, et al. The development and validation of an endoscopic grading system for Barrett's esophagus: the Prague C & M criteria. Gastroenterology 2006;131(5):1392–9.

33. Endoscopic Classification Review Group. Update on the Paris classification of superficial neoplastic lesions in the digestive tract. Endoscopy 2005;37(6):570–8.

34. Sharma P, Hawes RH, Bansal A, et al. Standard endoscopy with random biop-sies versus narrow band imaging targeted biopsies in Barrett's oesophagus: a prospective, international, randomised controlled trial. Gut 2012. [Epub ahead of print].

35. Sharma P, Meining AR, Coron E, et al. Real-time increased detection of neoplastic tissue in Barrett's esophagus with probe-based confocal laser endo-microscopy: final results of an international multicenter, prospective, random-ized, controlled trial. Gastrointest Endosc 2011;74(3):465–72.

36. Gaddam S, Mathur SC, Singh M, et al. Novel probe-based confocal laser endo-microscopy criteria and interobserver agreement for the detection of dysplasia in Barrett's esophagus. Am J Gastroenterol 2011;106(11):1961–9.

37. Gaddam S, Abrams JA, Coron E, et al. External validation of novel probe-based confocal laser endomicroscopy (pCLE) criteria for the diagnosis of dysplasia in Barrett's esophagus (BE). Gastroenterology 2011;140(5 Suppl 1):S-108.

38. Singh M, Mathur SC, Gaddam S, et al. Probe based confocal laser endomicro-scopy (pCLE) for the diagnosis of dysplasia in Barrett's esophagus (BE): accu-racy and interobserver agreement among gastrointestinal pathologists. Gastroenterology 2011;140(5 Suppl 1):S-186.

39. Young PE, Gentry AB, Acosta RD, et al. Endoscopic ultrasound does not accu-rately stage early adenocarcinoma or high-grade dysplasia of the esophagus. Clin Gastroenterol Hepatol 2010;8(12):1037–41.

40. Pouw RE, Heldoorn N, Herrero LA, et al. Do we still need EUS in the workup of patients with early esophageal neoplasia? A retrospective analysis of 131 cases. Gastrointest Endosc 2011;73(4):662–8.

41. Pech O, Gunter E, Dusemund F, et al. Accuracy of endoscopic ultrasound in preoperative staging of esophageal cancer: results from a referral center for early esophageal cancer. Endoscopy 2010;42(6):456–61.

42. May A, Gunter E, Roth F, et al. Accuracy of staging in early oesophageal cancer using high resolution endoscopy and high resolution endosonography: a comparative, prospective, and blinded trial. Gut 2004;53(5):634–40.

43. Chemaly M, Scalone O, Durivage G, et al. Miniprobe EUS in the pretherapeutic assessment of early esophageal neoplasia. Endoscopy 2008;40(1):2–6.

44. Wani SB, Edmundowicz SA, Abrams JA, et al. Accuracy of endoscopic ultrasonography (EUS) in staging early neoplasia in Barrett's esophagus (BE): results from a large multicenter cohort study. Gastrointest Endosc 2011;73(Suppl 4):AB166-7.

45. Prasad GA, Buttar NS, Wongkeesong LM, et al. Significance of neoplastic involvement of margins obtained by endoscopic mucosal resection in Barrett's esophagus. Am J Gastroenterol 2007;102(11):2380-6.

46. Chennat J, Konda VJ, Ross AS, et al. Complete Barrett's eradication endoscopic mucosal resection: an effective treatment modality for high-grade dysplasia and intramucosal carcinoma. An American single-center experience. Am J Gastroenterol 2009;104(11):2684-92.

47. Moss A, Bourke MJ, Hourigan LF, et al. Endoscopic resection for Barrett's high-grade dysplasia and early esophageal adenocarcinoma: an essential staging procedure with long-term therapeutic benefit. Am J Gastroenterol 2010; 105(6):1276-83.

48. Wani SB, Abrams JA, Edmundowicz SA, et al. Diagnostic endoscopic mucosal resection (EMR) leads to a change in histologic diagnosis in Barrett's esophagus (BE) patients with visible and flat neoplasia. Gastroenterology 2011; 140(5 Suppl 1):S-217-8.

49. Wani S, Mathur SC, Curvers WL, et al. Greater interobserver agreement by endoscopic mucosal resection than biopsy samples in Barrett's dysplasia. Clin Gastroenterol Hepatol 2010;8(9):783-8.

50. Pech O, Behrens A, May A, et al. Long-term results and risk factor analysis for recurrence after curative endoscopic therapy in 349 patients with high-grade intraepithelial neoplasia and mucosal adenocarcinoma in Barrett's oesophagus. Gut 2008;57(9):1200-6.

51. Shaheen NJ, Sharma P, Overholt BF, et al. Radiofrequency ablation in Barrett's esophagus with dysplasia. N Engl J Med 2009;360(22):2277-88.

52. Sharma VK, Wang KK, Overholt BF, et al. Balloon-based, circumferential, endoscopic radiofrequency ablation of Barrett's esophagus: 1-year follow-up of 100 patients. Gastrointest Endosc 2007;65(2):185-95.

53. Shaheen NJ, Overholt BF, Sampliner RE, et al. Durability of radiofrequency ablation in Barrett's esophagus with dysplasia. Gastroenterology 2011;141(2):460-8.

54. Fleischer DE, Overholt BF, Sharma VK, et al. Endoscopic radiofrequency ablation for Barrett's esophagus: 5-year outcomes from a prospective multicenter trial. Endoscopy 2010;42(10):781-9.

55. Tsai TH, Zhou C, Lee HC, et al. Comparison of tissue architectural changes between radiofrequency ablation and cryospray ablation in Barrett's esophagus using endoscopic three-dimensional optical coherence tomography. Gastroenterol Res Pract 2012. [Epub ahead of print].

56. Xue HB, Tan HH, Liu WZ, et al. A pilot study of endoscopic spray cryotherapy by pressurized carbon dioxide gas for Barrett's esophagus. Endoscopy 2011; 43(5):379-85.

57. Shaheen NJ, Greenwald BD, Peery AF, et al. Safety and efficacy of endoscopic spray cryotherapy for Barrett's esophagus with high-grade dysplasia. Gastrointest Endosc 2010;71(4):680-5.

58. Greenwald BD, Dumot JA, Horwhat JD, et al. Safety, tolerability, and efficacy of endoscopic low-pressure liquid nitrogen spray cryotherapy in the esophagus. Dis Esophagus 2010;23(1):13-9.

59. Dumot JA, Vargo JJ II, Falk GW, et al. An open-label, prospective trial of cryospray ablation for Barrett's esophagus high-grade dysplasia and early esophageal cancer in high-risk patients. Gastrointest Endosc 2009;70(4):635-44.

60. Pouw RE, van Vilsteren FG, Peters FP, et al. Randomized trial on endoscopic resection-cap versus multiband mucosectomy for piecemeal endoscopic resection of early Barrett's neoplasia. Gastrointest Endosc 2011;74(1):35–43.
61. van Vilsteren FG, Pouw RE, Seewald S, et al. Stepwise radical endoscopic resection versus radiofrequency ablation for Barrett's oesophagus with high-grade dysplasia or early cancer: a multicentre randomised trial. Gut 2011; 60(6):765–73.
62. Pouw RE, Seewald S, Gondrie JJ, et al. Stepwise radical endoscopic resection for eradication of Barrett's oesophagus with early neoplasia in a cohort of 169 patients. Gut 2010;59(9):1169–77.
63. Gerke H, Siddiqui J, Nasr I, et al. Efficacy and safety of EMR to completely remove Barrett's esophagus: experience in 41 patients. Gastrointest Endosc 2011;74(4):761–71.
64. Peters FP, Kara MA, Rosmolen WD, et al. Endoscopic treatment of high-grade dysplasia and early stage cancer in Barrett's esophagus. Gastrointest Endosc 2005;61(4):506–14.
65. May A, Gossner L, Pech O, et al. Local endoscopic therapy for intraepithelial high-grade neoplasia and early adenocarcinoma in Barrett's oesophagus: acute-phase and intermediate results of a new treatment approach. Eur J Gastroenterol Hepatol 2002;14(10):1085–91.
66. Ell C, May A, Gossner L, et al. Endoscopic mucosal resection of early cancer and high-grade dysplasia in Barrett's esophagus. Gastroenterology 2000; 118(4):670–7.
67. Soetikno RM, Gotoda T, Nakanishi Y, et al. Endoscopic mucosal resection. Gastrointest Endosc 2003;57(4):567–79.
68. Chung A, Bourke MJ, Hourigan LF, et al. Complete Barrett's excision by stepwise endoscopic resection in short-segment disease: long term outcomes and predictors of stricture. Endoscopy 2011;43(12):1025–32.
69. Katada C, Muto M, Manabe T, et al. Esophageal stenosis after endoscopic mucosal resection of superficial esophageal lesions. Gastrointest Endosc 2003;57(2):165–9.
70. Larghi A, Lightdale CJ, Ross AS, et al. Long-term follow-up of complete Barrett's eradication endoscopic mucosal resection (CBE-EMR) for the treatment of high grade dysplasia and intramucosal carcinoma. Endoscopy 2007;39(12):1086–91.
71. Lewis JJ, Rubenstein JH, Singal AG, et al. Factors associated with esophageal stricture formation after endoscopic mucosal resection for neoplastic Barrett's esophagus. Gastrointest Endosc 2011;74(4):753–60.
72. Pouw RE, Wirths K, Eisendrath P, et al. Efficacy of radiofrequency ablation combined with endoscopic resection for Barrett's esophagus with early neoplasia. Clin Gastroenterol Hepatol 2010;8(1):23–9.
73. Okoro NI, Tomizawa Y, Dunagan KT, et al. Safety of prior endoscopic mucosal resection in patients receiving radiofrequency ablation of Barrett's esophagus. Clin Gastroenterol Hepatol 2012;10(2):150–4.
74. Hvid-Jensen F, Pedersen L, Drewes AM, et al. Incidence of adenocarcinoma among patients with Barrett's esophagus. N Engl J Med 2011;365(15):1375–83.
75. Rastogi A, Puli S, El-Serag HB, et al. Incidence of esophageal adenocarcinoma in patients with Barrett's esophagus and high-grade dysplasia: a meta-analysis. Gastrointest Endosc 2008;67(3):394–8.
76. Wani S, Falk GW, Post J, et al. Risk factors for progression of low-grade dysplasia in patients with Barrett's esophagus. Gastroenterology 2011;141(4): 1179–86, 1186.e1.

77. Wani S. Management of low-grade dysplasia in Barrett's esophagus. Curr Opin Gastroenterol 2012;28(4):370–6.
78. Curvers WL, ten Kate FJ, Krishnadath KK, et al. Low-grade dysplasia in Barrett's esophagus: overdiagnosed and underestimated. Am J Gastroenterol 2010; 105(7):1523–30.
79. Srivastava A, Hornick JL, Li X, et al. Extent of low-grade dysplasia is a risk factor for the development of esophageal adenocarcinoma in Barrett's esophagus. Am J Gastroenterol 2007;102(3):483–93 [quiz: 694].
80. Lim CH, Treanor D, Dixon MF, et al. Low-grade dysplasia in Barrett's esophagus has a high risk of progression. Endoscopy 2007;39(7):581–7.
81. Dulai GS, Shekelle PG, Jensen DM, et al. Dysplasia and risk of further neoplastic progression in a regional Veterans Administration Barrett's cohort. Am J Gastroenterol 2005;100(4):775–83.
82. Conio M, Blanchi S, Lapertosa G, et al. Long-term endoscopic surveillance of patients with Barrett's esophagus. Incidence of dysplasia and adenocarcinoma: a prospective study. Am J Gastroenterol 2003;98(9):1931–9.
83. Schnell TG, Sontag SJ, Chejfec G, et al. Long-term nonsurgical management of Barrett's esophagus with high-grade dysplasia. Gastroenterology 2001;120(7): 1607–19.
84. Montgomery E, Bronner MP, Goldblum JR, et al. Reproducibility of the diagnosis of dysplasia in Barrett esophagus: a reaffirmation. Hum Pathol 2001;32(4):368–78.
85. Montes CG, Brandalise NA, Deliza R, et al. Antireflux surgery followed by bipolar electrocoagulation in the treatment of Barrett's esophagus. Gastrointest Endosc 1999;50(2):173–7.
86. Sampliner RE, Faigel D, Fennerty MB, et al. Effective and safe endoscopic reversal of nondysplastic Barrett's esophagus with thermal electrocoagulation combined with high-dose acid inhibition: a multicenter study. Gastrointest Endosc 2001;53(6):554–8.
87. Kelty CJ, Ackroyd R, Brown NJ, et al. Endoscopic ablation of Barrett's oesophagus: a randomized-controlled trial of photodynamic therapy vs. argon plasma coagulation. Aliment Pharmacol Ther 2004;20(11–12):1289–96.
88. Dulai GS, Jensen DM, Cortina G, et al. Randomized trial of argon plasma coagulation vs. multipolar electrocoagulation for ablation of Barrett's esophagus. Gastrointest Endosc 2005;61(2):232–40.
89. Madisch A, Miehlke S, Bayerdorffer E, et al. Long-term follow-up after complete ablation of Barrett's esophagus with argon plasma coagulation. World J Gastroenterol 2005;11(8):1182–6.
90. Manner H, May A, Miehlke S, et al. Ablation of nonneoplastic Barrett's mucosa using argon plasma coagulation with concomitant esomeprazole therapy (AP-BANEX): a prospective multicenter evaluation. Am J Gastroenterol 2006; 101(8):1762–9.
91. Sharma P, Wani S, Weston AP, et al. A randomised controlled trial of ablation of Barrett's oesophagus with multipolar electrocoagulation versus argon plasma coagulation in combination with acid suppression: long term results. Gut 2006;55(9):1233–9.
92. Mork H, Al-Taie O, Berlin F, et al. High recurrence rate of Barrett's epithelium during long-term follow-up after argon plasma coagulation. Scand J Gastroenterol 2007;42(1):23–7.
93. Fleischer DE, Overholt BF, Sharma VK, et al. Endoscopic ablation of Barrett's esophagus: a multicenter study with 2.5-year follow-up. Gastrointest Endosc 2008;68(5):867–76.

94. Bright T, Watson DI, Tam W, et al. Prospective randomized trial of argon plasma coagulation ablation versus endoscopic surveillance of Barrett's esophagus in patients treated with antisecretory medication. Dig Dis Sci 2009;54(12): 2606–11.

95. Hur C, Choi SE, Rubenstein JH, et al. The cost effectiveness of radiofrequency ablation for Barrett's esophagus. Gastroenterology 2012;143:567–75.

96. Falk GW. Radiofrequency ablation of Barrett's esophagus: let's not get ahead of ourselves. Dig Dis Sci 2010;55(7):1811–4.

97. Gupta N, Mathur SC, Dumot JA, et al. Adequacy of esophageal squamous mucosa specimens obtained during endoscopy: are standard biopsies sufficient for postablation surveillance in Barrett's esophagus? Gastrointest Endosc 2012;75(1):11–8.

98. Gray NA, Odze RD, Spechler SJ. Buried metaplasia after endoscopic ablation of Barrett's esophagus: a systematic review. Am J Gastroenterol 2011;106(11): 1899–908 [quiz: 1909].

99. Wani S, Sayana H, Sharma P. Endoscopic eradication of Barrett's esophagus. Gastrointest Endosc 2010;71(1):147–66.

100. Lyday WD, Corbett FS, Kuperman DA, et al. Radiofrequency ablation of Barrett's esophagus: outcomes of 429 patients from a multicenter community practice registry. Endoscopy 2010;42(4):272–8.

101. Wani S, Puli SR, Shaheen NJ, et al. Esophageal adenocarcinoma in Barrett's esophagus after endoscopic ablative therapy: a meta-analysis and systematic review. Am J Gastroenterol 2009;104(2):502–13.

102. Hernandez JC, Reicher S, Chung D, et al. Pilot series of radiofrequency ablation of Barrett's esophagus with or without neoplasia. Endoscopy 2008;40(5): 388–92.

103. Van Laethem JL, Peny MO, Salmon I, et al. Intramucosal adenocarcinoma arising under squamous re-epithelialisation of Barrett's oesophagus. Gut 2000;46(4):574–7.

104. Titi M, Overhiser A, Ulusarac O, et al. Development of subsquamous high-grade dysplasia and adenocarcinoma after successful radiofrequency ablation of Barrett's esophagus. Gastroenterology 2012;143(3):564–566.e1.

105. Zhou C, Tsai TH, Lee HC, et al. Characterization of buried glands before and after radiofrequency ablation by using 3-dimensional optical coherence tomography (with videos). Gastrointest Endosc 2012;76(1):32–40.

106. Peery AF, Shaheen NJ. Optical coherence tomography in Barrett's esophagus: the road to clinical utility. Gastrointest Endosc 2010;71(2):231–4.

107. Cobb MJ, Hwang JH, Upton MP, et al. Imaging of subsquamous Barrett's epithelium with ultrahigh-resolution optical coherence tomography: a histologic correlation study. Gastrointest Endosc 2010;71(2):223–30.

108. Adler DC, Zhou C, Tsai TH, et al. Three-dimensional optical coherence tomography of Barrett's esophagus and buried glands beneath neosquamous epithelium following radiofrequency ablation. Endoscopy 2009;41(9):773–6.

Advances in Endoluminal Therapy for Esophageal Cancer

Brintha K. Enestvedt, MD, MBA[a],*, Gregory G. Ginsberg, MD[b]

KEYWORDS

- Endoscopic therapy • Early esophageal cancer • Superficial esophageal cancer
- Endoscopic mucosal resection • Endoscopic submucosal dissection
- Mucosal ablation • Self-expanding metal stents • Palliation of esophageal cancer

KEY POINTS

- Advances in endoscopic therapy have resulted in dramatic changes in the way early esophageal cancer is managed and in the palliation of dysphagia related to advanced esophageal cancer.
- Endoscopic mucosal resection (EMR) and endoscopic submucosal dissection (ESD) are effective therapies for accurate histopathologic staging and provide a potential for complete cure.
- Mucosal ablative techniques are effective adjuncts to EMR and ESD and reduce the occurrence of synchronous and metachronous lesions within the Barrett esophagus.
- These techniques have placed the endoscopist at the multidisciplinary table in discussions of management of esophageal cancer, rather than solely being the diagnostician as in the past.
- Self-expanding metal stents (SEMS) has anchored itself as a durable and immediate modality for the relief of malignant dysphagia from esophageal cancer.

INTRODUCTION

Esophageal cancer is diagnosed in approximately 400,000 patients a year, but its true incidence has been challenging to estimate given the possibility of misclassifying gastroesophageal (GE) junction esophageal cancers as gastric cardia cancers. For all patients with esophageal cancer, the 5-year survival is approximately 20% or less. Given this strikingly poor prognosis, early detection and treatment offers the most promising prospect for improved survival or potentially even cure.

Financial disclosures: None.
[a] Division of Gastroenterology, Temple University, 3401 North Broad Street, Parkinson Pavilion, 8th Floor, Philadelphia, PA 19140, USA; [b] Division of Gastroenterology, University of Pennsylvania, 3400 Spruce Street, Philadelphia, PA 19104, USA
* Corresponding author.
E-mail address: brintha.e@gmail.com

Esophageal cancers are characterized as squamous cell carcinoma or adenocarcinoma, the latter arising in association with Barrett esophagus. In the Western world, esophageal adenocarcinoma has surpassed squamous cell carcinoma as the predominant esophageal malignancy. These 2 cancer types differ in their rates of lymph node metastases. Lymph node metastases can be seen in up to 10% of patients with mucosal squamous cell tumors and in 50% of those with submucosal invasion. On the contrary, lymph node metastases are uncommon in patients with early esophageal adenocarcinoma. Independent of the type of esophageal cancer, endoluminal therapies are stratified into therapy for early-stage esophageal cancer and palliation of dysphagia symptoms in patients with metastatic disease or locally unresectable disease. Early esophageal cancers are those classified as Tis or high-grade dysplasia (HGD) (formerly called carcinoma in situ) or T1 tumors (involvement limited to the mucosa or submucosa).

Endoscopic therapies for early esophageal cancer continue to evolve. Advances in endoscopic technologies and techniques such as enhanced mucosal imaging, endoscopic ultrasound (EUS), and EMR have allowed for improved early cancer detection, staging, and eradication. It is imperative, however, to incorporate advanced endoscopic therapeutics for esophageal cancers in the context of a multidisciplinary setting to include surgical, medical, and radiation oncology expertise.

Endoscopic therapy for esophageal cancer can be stratified into management of early esophageal cancer (superficial cancers) and palliation of advanced cancer. This article begins with a brief review of the past management of early esophageal cancer, namely, esophagectomy and then reviews the available endoluminal therapies including EMR, ESD, thermal laser, argon plasma coagulation (APC), photodynamic therapy (PDT), and cryotherapy. Finally, this article reviews endoluminal palliative options, namely, endoprosthetics (SEMS).

MANAGEMENT OF EARLY ESOPHAGEAL CANCER
Operative Resection

The optimal treatment approach for patients with localized esophageal cancer remains controversial as new less-invasive endoscopic technology emerges to challenge traditional surgical esophagectomy. Before the emergence of advanced endoscopic techniques, esophagectomy was the treatment of choice for patients with localized squamous cell carcinoma, adenocarcinoma, intramucosal carcinoma (ImCa), and multifocal HGD in association with Barrett esophagus.[1] Both transhiatal and transthoracic esophagectomy are frequently performed in the United States without a clear 5-year survival benefit of one over the other as reported from 2 large outcomes databases[2,3]; however, transhiatal esophagectomy is generally preferred in those with T1 cancers, based on its reduced morbidity (pulmonary complications, chylothorax, blood loss, shorter intensive care unit and hospital stay).[4,5] In general, 5-year survival rates for esophagectomy for early esophageal cancer ranges from 63% to 83%. It is now clearly recognized that the outcomes of esophagectomy are a function of hospital and surgical volumes.[6,7] At high-volume centers, the mortality associated with esophagectomy may be 2% (range of 0%–5%), but morbidity rates remain high, ranging from 30% to 50%. The introduction of a minimally invasive laparoscopic transhiatal approach (combined thorascopic–laparoscopic) seems to be associated with lower perioperative morbidity and mortality and may lead to improved overall survival and disease-free survival in expert hands.[8–11]

The morbidity and mortality associated with surgical esophagectomy and the low rates of metastases associated with early esophageal cancer have led to the interest in local endoscopic therapy as an alternative to surgery. Few data are available directly comparing the surgical and endoscopic management of early esophageal cancer and what exists are retrospective and observational. The available literature suggests that long-term outcomes including median cancer-free survival with endoscopic therapy for early esophageal cancer is similar to that of surgical therapy with fewer complications, but a higher rate of recurrence.[12–14] A recognized drawback of endoscopic monotherapy for early esophageal cancer in Barrett esophagus is the rate of recurrence (which can be as high as 22% in some series).[15] However, the most recurrences can be endoscopically salvaged and do not lead to death from disease. These data suggest that endoscopic therapy can be used in intramucosal esophageal cancer with oncologic outcomes equivalent to surgery.

Staging

The overall outcome of esophageal cancer is strongly associated with its stage, therefore accurate staging is critical to providing estimations of prognosis and appropriate selection of treatment. **Table 1** contains the T category definitions for esophageal cancer (both squamous cell and adenocarcinoma) and includes a more comprehensive subclassification scheme proposed for early esophageal cancers. **Fig. 1** contains a graphical representation of the depth of invasion of esophageal tumors and their risk of lymph node metastases.[28] Overall, mucosal-based lesions are associated with very low rates of lymph node metastases (<3%); however, tumors that invade the submucosa have a substantial risk of lymph node metastases. In general, esophageal cancer staging involves a multimodal approach including computed tomography (CT), fludeoxyglucose F18 positron emission tomography (FDG-PET), and EUS. After diagnosis, staging usually begins with a CT scan of the chest and abdomen to evaluate for distant metastatic disease. CT, however, has poor sensitivity for celiac lymph nodes and small metastases (particular peritoneal metastases) and cannot reliably assess for depth of tumor invasion.[29] FDG-PET scans have improved sensitivity for small metastases and are routinely used in preoperative staging when traditional CT

Table 1
T category definitions for esophageal cancer

Tx	Primary tumor cannot be assessed	
T0	No evidence of primary tumor	
Tis, m1	High-grade dysplasia, limited to mucosal layer	
T1	Tumor invades lamina propria, muscularis mucosa or submucosa	T1a
T1, m2	Tumor invades the lamina propria	
T1, m3	Tumor invades into but not through the muscularis mucosa	T1b
T1, sm1	Tumor invades into the shallowest one-third of the submucosa	
T1, sm2	Tumor invades into the intermediate one-third of the submucosa	
T1, sm3	Tumor penetrates the deepest one-third of the submucosa	
T2	Tumor invades the muscularis propria	
T3	Tumor invades adventitia	
T4	Tumor invades adjacent structures	
T4a	Resectable tumor that invades pleura, pericardiam, or diaphragm	
T4b	Unresectable tumor invading aorta, vertebra, tracea, or other adjacent structures	

Adapted from Edge SB, Byyrd DR, Compton CC, et al. American Joint Committee on Cancer Staging manual. 7th edition. New York: Springer; 2010. p. 103; with permission.

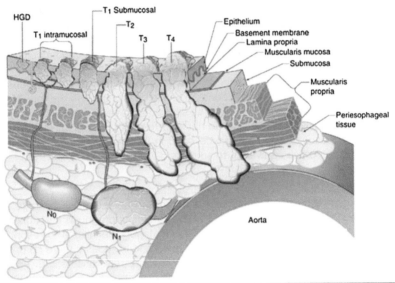

Depth of lesion	HGD	T1a m2	T1a m3	T1b sm1	T1b sm2	T1b sm3
Risk of lymph node metastasis*	0%	0–6%	0–12%	8–32%	12–28%	20–67%

Fig. 1. Depth of tumor invasion and risk of lymph node metastases. The asterisk indicates that percentages are aggregated from multiple studies[16–27] of adenocarcinoma and squamous cell carcinoma. (*From* Rice WR: Diagnosis and staging of esophageal carcinoma. In Pearson FG, Cooper JD, Deslauriers J, et al [eds]: Esophageal Surgery, 2nd ed. New York: Churchill Livingstone; 2002. p. 687; with permission.)

demonstrates no distant disease; however, it too has poor sensitivity and specificity for locoregional disease staging.

EUS and EMR have allowed for more precise assessments of tumor depth and likelihood of regional lymph node metastases. In the past, early esophageal cancer was defined by the endoscopic criteria diameter less than or equal to 2 cm. However, this method clearly was unable to predict the depth of invasion or local lymph node involvement. At that time, only surgery was able to provide these additional assessments. These surgical resections have revealed that early esophageal cancers, those that do not penetrate the muscularis mucosa, are rarely associated with metastatic disease.[16,30,31]

The development of EUS has obviated surgical T staging of esophageal cancer. EUS allows the endoscopist to visualize at 7.5 to 12.5 MHz transducer frequencies to delineate lesions and their depth of penetration into or through the 5-layer esophageal wall pattern. It also enables examination of periesophageal, celiac, and perigastric lymph nodes (all N1 categories) as well as most of the liver (M1 category), pleura, and vascular structures (T4 stage). Suspicious-appearing lymph nodes—those that are hypoechoic, round, in proximity to the tumor, and greater than 1 cm in diameter—may be sampled using the linear array echoendoscope for EUS-guided fine-needle aspiration. Higher-frequency probes that image at 20 to 30 MHz can image mucosal lesions at a higher resolution, if deemed necessary. These probes also eliminate artifact caused by compression of the endosonographic balloon that is traditionally used with EUS. However, higher-frequency EUS probes are limited by lack of deep tissue visualization. In most cases, traditional EUS (without the use of higher-frequency probes) is sufficient to stage esophageal cancer. Studies have demonstrated that preoperative staging by EUS performed at high-volume EUS centers (>50 EUS/endoscopist/year) is more sensitive and specific than when performed at low-volume centers.[29] Therefore, EUS should be performed by experienced endosonographers to optimize patient selection for esophageal resection. EUS is considered the most accurate available locoregional staging modality, with an accuracy of 80% to 90% of T and N staging,[32,33] whereas some data suggest that its accuracy is diminished to approximately 65% for superficial T1 cancers[34] and that it cannot reliably differentiate between T1a and T1b lesions. On the contrary, a meta-analysis (19 studies) shows that EUS is accurate for staging of T1a and T1b tumors.[35] The accuracy of EUS may be influenced by the experience of the endosonographer. Differentiating mucosal lesions from those that infiltrate the submucosa is much more difficult in the setting of Barrett esophagus than in squamous cell carcinoma given that crypts and villi in Barrett esophagus are more heterogeneous than the layered architecture of squamous epithelium. Barrett esophagous tends to be associated with more inflammatory changes that result in a double muscularis mucosae, and Barrett-esophagus-related neoplasms tend to be located close to the cardia, which is a difficult area for EUS interpretation. Some studies infer that there is limited added value of EUS for determining T category once tumor depth has been estimated by expert endoscopic inspection.[36] Most authorities now, however, agree that histopathologic inspection of the suspected lesion obtained by endoscopic resection is now considered the most accurate means to assess the depth of tumor infiltration (pathologic T category) and the risk of lymph node involvement.

EMR has emerged as a diagnostic, staging, and therapeutic technique. This technique provides a greater volume of tissue for diagnostic purposes. The specimen yields the most accurate T staging for superficial esophageal cancers. Most importantly, for lesions confined to the mucosa and in certain cases the submucosa, it can be curative. At present, EMR is the standard therapy for treatment of early esophageal cancer in association with Barrett esophagus. Various techniques of EMR are discussed separately in the following sections.

Endoscopic Resection

Historically, surgery was considered the modality of choice for early esophageal cancer including ImCa and HGD in the setting of Barrett esophagus. Although cure rates were very high, they came at the cost of treatment-related morbidity and mortality. Given the very low risk of lymph node metastases associated with these conditions and the reported morbidity (30%–40%) and mortality (2%–5%) associated with esophagectomy (at high-volume centers performing >20 operations a year),[6,7] endoluminal eradication and ablative therapies have surpassed surgery as the modality of choice. The goals of endoscopic therapy are to preserve the esophagus while achieving curative eradication. EMR, ESD, and mucosal ablative techniques including radiofrequency ablation (RFA), thermal laser therapy, APC, and PDT are discussed in the following sections.

Endoscopic mucosal resection (EMR)

EMR is an extension of standard snare polypectomy for the eradication of mucosal-based lesions that may not otherwise be amenable to endoscopic resection. Although the intent is often curative, it is used for enhanced diagnostic and staging purposes. EMR is also referred to as mucosectomy or endoluminal resection. The major advantage of EMR is that it delivers a large specimen, which provides a more accurate histologic diagnosis given the increased depth and volume of tissue sampling compared with standard biopsy forceps. **Fig. 2** exemplifies a nodular lesion and the defect created after EMR. HGD and T1a tumors (m2 and m3) are the most appropriate candidate lesions for endoscopic resection given that lymph node metastasis is extremely rare.

When feasible, EMR is highly successful in achieving cure rates for HGD and ImCa in association with Barrett esophagus, with up to 96% complete response at a mean follow-up of 63 months in the largest observation series.[15] The same series demonstrated that a significant drawback of EMR cure was the high rate of recurrent or metachronous lesions during follow-up, approaching 22%. Most of these patients can be adequately salvaged with endoscopic therapy alone, rather than surgery or death.[12,13,37] Although no randomized controlled trial exists, the available literature demonstrates that there is no apparent difference in long-term outcomes (long-term complete response and overall survival) between EMR and surgery for early esophageal cancer.[12–14]

There are several techniques available for EMR: cap-assisted, ligation-assisted, and injection-assisted EMR.[38,39] The most commonly used techniques are the ligation-assisted and cap-assisted EMR. Irrespective of the EMR technique, before resection, a thorough white light and electronically enhanced (eg, narrow band imaging) examination is critical to identify and characterize suspect surface abnormalities. In order to sustain visibility of the targeted area for resection, the borders of the lesion may be marked using a cautery device such as multipolar coagulator (ie, tip of the snare).

Cap-assisted EMR Cap-assisted EMR uses a transparent cap fitted over the tip of the endoscope. The lesion is lifted with a submucosal injection of saline or diluted epinephrine, and the cap is subsequently centered over the lesion and suction is applied to retract the lesion into the cap. A preseated snare is then immediately closed to capture the neopolypoid tissue, and suction is then released. The lesion is then snare-resected with electrocautery (**Fig. 3B**). This application is particularly useful for flat or nodular lesions. The cap is available in a completely flat, level lip, or an obliquely angulated cap end. The straight flat cap is favored when precision is required in the amount of tissue necessary for resection, whereas the oblique cap allows for larger resections. This technique was pioneered in Japan, where EMR is the standard of care for superficial esophageal cancer.

Ligation-assisted EMR Ligation-assisted EMR or multiband mucosectomy uses a modified band ligation system similar to that of variceal band ligation. The endoscope is fitted with a friction cap that attaches to the tip of a standard or therapeutic

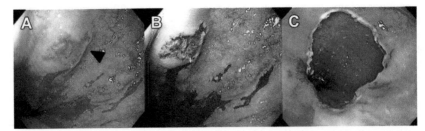

Fig. 2. Nodular lesion and defect after piecemeal wide-area endoscopic mucosal resection. (A) Nodular lesion visible on high-definition white light endoscopy and narrow band imaging. (B, C) Endoscopic appearance after piecemeal wide-area endoscopic mucosal resection (ligation-assisted EMR was performed).

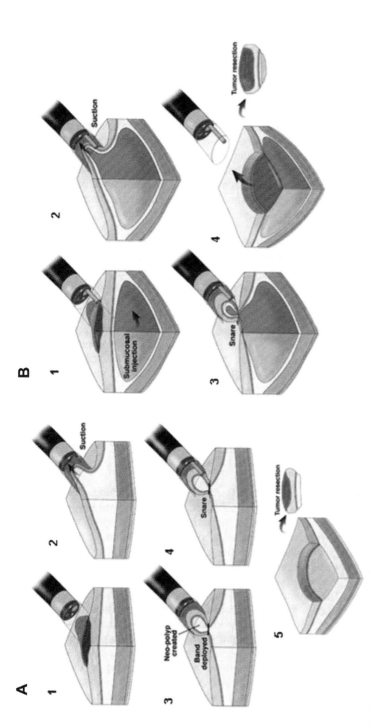

Fig. 3. Ligation-assisted and cap-assisted endoscopic mucosa resection. (A) Ligation-assisted EMR involves the use of a transparent cap affixed to the tip of the endoscope, modified with a band ligation system. The tip of the endoscope is positioned over the target tissue (1) and suction is applied and the lesion drawn up into the banding chamber (2). A band is deployed entrapping the tissue and creating a neopolyp (3). The neopolyp is then resected using electrocautery snare technique applied below, above, or through the band (4), leaving a well demarginated mucosal defect at the resection site (5). (B) Cap-assisted EMR involves the use of a transparent cap that is fitted over the tip of the endoscope. After submucosal injection beneath the target lesion (1), the cap is centered over the lesion and suction is used to retract the lesion up and into the cap (2). A preseated snare is then closed to capture the neopolypoid tissue (3), and suction is released. The ensnared tissue is then resected with application of electrocautery (4). (From Chandrasekhara V, Ginsberg GG. Endoscopic mucosal resection: not your father's polypectomy anymore. Gastroenterology 2011;141(1):42–9; with permission.)

endoscope. The cap is used to suction the target lesion into the banding chamber. A band is deployed, entrapping the tissue and thereby creating a neopolyp. The neopolyp is then resected using snare electrocautery below, above, or through the band (see **Fig. 3**A). Some endoscopists use preligation submucosal injection to lift the mucosal-based lesion away from the musclaris propria and provide an elevated purchase around which a snare can be placed. This ligation-assisted EMR technique is attractive because the band routinely extrudes the muscularis propria layer entrapping only the mucosa and portions of the submucosa. Second, the system allows efficient repeated applications to enable wide-area confluent resections during a single session. The average diameter of the resected mucosa is approximately 15 mm when assessed by pathologists. A multiband mucosectomy device is commercially available (Duette; Cook Medical, Limerick, Ireland) for use with high-definition and therapeutic channel endoscopes. A prospective study of 243 procedures with a total of 1060 resections performed with ligation-assisted technique demonstrated complete resection in 91% with low rates of complication (bleeding in 3%, no perforations).[40]

Ligation-assisted EMR has several advantages: (1) it does not require submucosal injection as with the cap-assisted technique because the muscularis propria will immediately retract when captured with a rubber band, whereas it may remain captured within the forcefully closed resection snare with cap-assisted EMR; (2) repeated withdrawal of the endoscope is not necessary with ligation-assisted EMR because the multiband device allows for 6 consecutive resections, thereby reducing cost and time; and (3) prelooping of the endoscopic resection snare in the ridge of the cap, which can be challenging, is not necessary. A randomized control trial of 84 patients compared cap-assisted EMR with ligation-assisted EMR[41] for piecemeal resection of early cancer in association with Barrett esophagus. The ligation-assisted technique had significantly shorter procedure times (34 minutes vs 50 minutes) and was less costly than cap-assisted EMR. There was no difference in the depth of resection between the 2 techniques. A total of 3 perforations occurred in the cap-assisted group compared with 1 in the ligation-assisted EMR cohort. The time and cost savings of ligation-assisted EMR may be borne in the fact that preresection submucosal lift is not required and a single snare may be used for all resections.

Injection-assisted EMR Injection-assisted EMR is akin to saline-assisted polypectomy of the colon. A solution is injected into the submucosal layer beneath the lesion to create a mound of tissue more suitable for ensnarement. This maneuver lifts the mucosal-based lesion away from the muscularis propria. Furthermore, the lift also reduces the electrosurgical resistance during snare resection with cautery. Injection-assisted EMR allows for resection of broad areas of tissue while minimizing the risk of perforation or transmural burn syndrome by protecting the muscularis propria with a saline cushion. The volume of fluid injected into the submucosa varies based on the lesion size and location. Although an ideal submucosal injectate remains to be determined, an admixture of methylene blue and normal saline solution is commonly used to aid in assessment of the lateral margins of the lesion and completeness and depth of resection. Some investigators also add diluted epinephrine to the injectate to reduce "back-bleeding" from the needle insertion and acute bleeding postresection.

Characteristics that are considered favorable for successful EMR are diameter less than 2 cm (for en bloc resection); lack of penetration of the muscularis mucosa; polypoid, flat, or elevated lesions; and well-differentiated histology (**Table 2**). Ulcerated or depressed lesions are less likely to demonstrate appropriate lifting and are therefore not favorable for EMR. Lesions larger than 2 cm can be resected in

Table 2	
Favorable esophageal cancer characteristics for endoscopic mucosal resection	
Characteristic	Favorable Outcome
Size	<2 cm
Depth of penetration	Muscularis mucosae is preserved
Grade of cancer	Well-differentiated cancer
Appearance	Elevated, polypoid, or flat

a piecemeal manner to achieve wide-area confluent mucosal resection, but care must be taken to sufficiently overlap areas of resection so that small neoplastic residues are not left behind. Therefore, if possible, en bloc resection allows for the most accurate lateral and deep margin histologic evaluation.

In summary, if endoscopy with or without EUS identifies only the mucosal extent of neoplasia, then the patient is appropriate for initiation of endoscopic therapy. Curative EMR is determined by the depth of invasion precisely assessed at histopathologic inspection of the resected specimen. The final path of the EMR specimen, including tumor grade, depth of invasion, presence or absence of tumor at the resection margins, and lymphovascular invasion, ultimately determines whether endoscopic therapy alone is adequate or operative resection is indicated. If EUS demonstrates that the esophageal cancer invades beyond the muscularis mucosa or if there is evidence of pathologic lymph nodes, operative resection is recommended in fit candidates. An alternative school of thought to the above-mentioned algorithm supports the use of EMR for T staging without concomitant EUS,[41] given the limitations of EUS in differentiating between T1a and T1b lesions. This practice, which the authors advocate, involves performing EMR for any endoscopically apparent superficial esophageal cancer with or without routine EUS examination.

Endoscopic submucosal dissection (ESD)
ESD was developed and popularized in Asia to obtain larger resected specimens en bloc with potential for complete excision of neoplastic lesions. ESD was initially described for the treatment of early gastric cancers in the stomach in Japan[42] but is used in many parts of Asia for endoscopic therapy for early esophageal cancers.

The first step in ESD is to mark the area targeted for resection usually by using cautery to ensure optimal visualization after submucosal injection and to ensure that at least a 3-mm margin is resected.[38] A submucosal bleb is formed in a manner similar to that described for EMR except that different injectates are commonly used. For ESD, a more durably persistent solution is used, given the approximate procedure duration of 1 to 2 hours. Examples of injectates include sodium hyaluronate, docium hydroxypropyl methylcellulose, sodium carboxymethylcellulose, hypertonic dextrose, hypertonic saline, or fibrinogen.[38] Once the entire specimen has been lifted with the submucosal injectate, the lesion is usually circumscribed with one or more specialized electrosurgical "knives" to isolate the lesion from the normal surrounding mucosa. The submucosal layer beneath the isolated lesion is then meticulously dissected with electrosurgical devices to be removed en bloc; this part of the procedure is the most challenging and requires expert control and skill.

Multiple ESD cutting accessories have been developed. The devices have considerable variations and are championed by various enthusiasts, and some are best suited for certain portions of the procedure. Several ESD knives are depicted in **Fig. 4.**

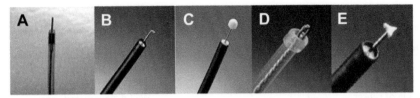

Fig. 4. Examples of knives for endoscopic submucosal dissection. (A) Needle knife, (B) HookKnife, (C) TT knife, (D) FlexKnife, (E) IT knife. (Images *courtesy of* Olympus.)

ESD, similar to EMR, provides pathologic staging and is intended for cure. EMR and ESD for the treatment of early esophageal cancer have been compared in a retrospective manner, and ESD was found to increase the cure rate for early squamous cell cancer from 71% to 97%.[43] However, for cancers less than 1.5 cm, there was no difference in the cure rate between ESD and EMR. This result was mirrored for early gastric cancer as well, with 1.5 cm representing a cutoff between the 2 techniques with similar cure rates and complications.[44]

Compared with EMR, ESD requires significant expertise. Training in ESD is a much more substantial undertaking than most other endoscopic therapeutic adoptions. Each procedure itself requires several hours to complete. However, the potential for larger en bloc specimens than EMR is appealing. Although ESD is performed in some Asian countries, its use at present is limited to the United States.

Endoscopic Ablation Therapies

Ablation techniques are intended to destroy target tissue to a relatively precise depth and breadth. As they do not provide a histopathologic specimen, they are largely considered suboptimal to resection therapies. However, some ablation therapies can be applied to broader areas and to lesion locations and characteristics that would prove not amenable to endoscopic resection. Such therapies include RFA, thermal laser, PDT, APC, and cryotherapy.

Radiofrequency ablation

RFA is used to ablate dysplastic and nondysplastic Barrett epithelium that entails the use of a balloon-based circumferential device (HALO360, Covidien, Sunnyvale, CA, USA) or a focal targeted device (HALO90, HALO60, HALO90 Ultra) for delivering a standardized amount of high-powered radiofrequency energy to designated tissues to achieve mucosal destruction without damaging the underlying muscularis propria. At present, the main indication is flat Barrett esophagus with HGD and eradication of the residual Barrett esophagus that contained nodular HGD or ImCa after EMR of the visible lesion.

The ablation technique has been developed to achieve reliable, precise, and uniform depth of ablation between 500 and 1000 μm. There are 2 delivery systems available: a 3-cm-long electrode on a 360° balloon catheter (HALO360) intended for confluent and circumferential segments and an endoscope-mounted articulating electrode platform intended for focal or short-length targeted segments (HALO90, HALO60, HALO90 Ultra) (Fig. 5). The technique involves mucosal ablation under endoscopic guidance followed by removal of the adhered coagulum in the ablated zone followed by repeat treatment within the same endoscopic session. The technical learning curve for RFA is small, and this technique is increasingly used in both academic and community practices with low complication rates.

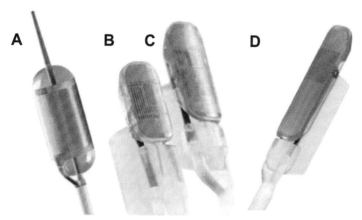

Fig. 5. Devices for radiofrequency ablation. (*A*) Balloon-based catheter (HALO360, 3-cm-long circumferential electrode), (*B*) HALO60 ablation catheter (15 mm length × 10 mm width electrode), (*C*) HALO90 ablation catheter (20 mm length × 13 mm width electrode), (*D*) HALO90 Ultra ablation catheter (40 mm length × 13 mm width electrode). (Images *courtesy of* BARRX Medical/Covidien.)

There have been multiple studies in the past several years that have consistently shown that RFA is a safe, effective, and well-tolerated therapy for dysplastic Barrett esophagus, with dysplasia eradication in up to 80% to 90% of patients and eradication of intestinal metaplasia in up to 95% of those with prior dysplasia.[45–48] The results are compelling, and RFA provides a safe and cost-effective alternative to surgery or surveillance in the management of dysplastic Barrett esophagus. In many settings, RFA is also being used for eradication in patients with low-grade dysplasia. RFA for *nondysplastic* Barrett esophagus remains controversial. Some pose that any Barrett esophagus represents a threat and therefore should be eradicated. On the contrary, others argue that eradication of nondysplastic Barrett esophagus is not cost effective given the very low rates of progression to esophageal adenocarcinoma and as such is prohibitively expensive from a public policy standpoint.[49–51]

As we gain more experience and longer follow-up with RFA, the development of subsquamous recurrence of dysplasia or even ImCa ("buried" Barrett esophagus) after ablation is a real and alarming concern.[52] Identification of such cases underscores the importance of continued and vigilant surveillance after RFA, even after complete eradication of intestinal metaplasia. It also emphasizes the need to use caution regarding the extensive use of RFA, especially in patients with low-risk Barrett esophagus.

RFA is often used as an adjunct therapy to localized EMR for management of early esophageal cancer associated with Barrett esophagus. Owing to the frequent multifocal HGD or ImCa within a field of Barrett epithelium, RFA is used to eradicate the residual Barrett esophagus to prevent synchronous and metachronous lesions. As such, nodular HGD or ImCa should be treated with EMR first, followed by RFA, to eradicate the residual dysplastic tissue or intestinal metaplasia given the risk of these tissues to progress to more advanced condition. It is worthwhile noting that nodular or endoscopically visible lesions associated with Barrett esophagus should not be treated with RFA alone. Studies have demonstrated that combined endoscopic therapy with EMR and RFA is indeed safe[53,54] with relatively similar rates of stricture formation in the EMR plus RFA group in comparison with the RFA alone group.

Thermal laser

Lasers differ in their wavelength and therefore the depth of penetration. Three types of lasers are available and operate at different wavelengths: the neodymium:yttrium-aluminum-garnet (Nd:YAG) laser (λ 1064 nm, 4 mm depth of penetration), potassium titanyl phosphate laser (λ 532 nm, 1 mm depth of penetration), and argon laser (λ 514.5 nm, 1 mm depth of penetration).

In the past, laser treatment was primarily used for palliation of advanced esophageal cancer. Although lasers were previously helpful in initial tumor ablation to increase the diameter of an obstructed esophageal lumen, they were costly and required several applications to achieve palliation and therefore became less desirable than SEMS. There had been some interest in the use of laser therapy for the treatment of superficial esophageal cancer and HGD. However, these studies had very few patients, and thus the efficacy experience was limited.[55–57] This technology has been largely supplanted by the use of expandable metal stents for palliation, and it is unlikely that lasers will have a role in the future treatment of early esophageal cancer.

Argon plasma coagulation (APC)

APC is a noncontact monopolar current transmitted to tissue via flow of ionized argon gas. The depth of penetration is approximately 6 mm and can vary depending on the generator power setting, gas flow, duration of application, and proximity of probe tip to the target tissue. APC was originally developed as a hemostatic technique, and because of its superficial effect, it has been regarded to have a decreased risk of perforation. Mucosal ablation with APC for Barrett esophagus has been studied with positive overall outcomes.[58–61] Overall, the experience with APC for superficial esophageal cancer is limited to a few small case series.[61,62] These case series demonstrate that complication rates are low and that failure rates of cancer eradication is higher with squamous cell cancer than Barrett-associated adenocarcinoma. The role of APC for early esophageal cancer in the current era of EMR, ESD, and RFA is uncertain.

Photodynamic therapy (PDT)

PDT takes advantage of drug–light interaction to induce cell death. First, a photosensitizing agent is administered to the patient hours to days before light delivery to allow time for the photosensitizing agent to concentrate in the tumor. After a specific time frame, the tumor cells that have retained the photosensitizing agent are exposed to wavelength-specific laser light that is delivered through a fiber through the endoscope channel. A light-induced toxic reaction ensues and results in targeted cell death.

PDT is approved for therapy for Barrett esophagus with HGD. PDT has been studied in the treatment of esophageal cancer. Several studies combine patients with advanced and early cancers. Although the numbers of patients are small, the results are impressive with 5-year survival rates between 74% and 93% for T0 or T1 cancers.[63–68] Most of these studies are relatively dated, and PDT has not been rigorously compared with EMR and RFA.

The largest drawback of PDT is the lack of a pathologic specimen. In addition, there is the potential for inadequate treatment leading to recurrence. Patients can experience numerous adverse events including cutaneous photosensitivity after drug administration, chest pain, odynophagia and nausea after photoradiation, dehydration, and esophageal strictures (occurring in approximately 1 of 3 patients treated with PDT and often requiring multiple endoscopic sessions to remediate). Given the potential adverse events and the lack of pathologic staging with PDT, it is not used at present in isolation for the treatment of early esophageal cancer; however, it may play a role in the future in combination with EMR for cancer eradication or in specific subsets of patients.

Cryotherapy

Cryotherapy is a relatively novel and evolving technology for endoscopic therapy of superficial esophageal cancer. While experience remains limited, preliminary results seem promising.[69] At present, 2 commercially developed cryotherapy systems are in use. One is performed with endoscopic spray of low-pressure liquid nitrogen, resulting in freezing of a segment of mucosa. Several cycles of freezing and thawing are performed at each site before proceeding to the next targeted area. Usually, several sessions of cryotherapy are required for complete local tumor eradication. The other system uses pressurized carbon dioxide.

Thus far, experience in the use of cryotherapy for early esophageal cancer is limited by a single series of 79 patients and lack of long-term follow-up.[69] These patients were enrolled at 10 different academic centers, and all had refused, failed, or were ineligible for conventional therapy for esophageal cancer. The cohort included all T categories of esophageal cancer (T1: 60 patients, T2: 16 patients, T3/4: 3 patients). Of the 79 patients, 49 completed the treatment protocol for cryotherapy. At a median of 10 months of follow-up, complete regression of disease was reported in 75% of those with mucosal cancer. However, recurrence of HGD after cryotherapy has been reported to be as high as 30% at 6 months.[70]

Cryotherapy is currently available and is being selectively used for treatment of Barrett dysplasia and early esophageal cancer. However, more data are necessary to help define its role in the current algorithmic approach to early esophageal cancer.

Endoscopic Therapy: Summary

In appropriately selected patients with T1a cancers, endoscopic therapy is highly effective and safe. EMR and ESD are highly desirable because they not only provide histopathologic staging but also have the potential for cure for early esophageal cancer. Multiple mucosal ablative techniques exist, and at present, they are generally used as adjunct to EMR in the treatment of disease related to Barrett esophagus. A large cohort analysis using this approach with long-term follow-up reported that 166 patients were treated and had at least 1 year of follow-up.[71] Complete elimination of neoplasia was achieved in 157 patients (95%) and complete elimination of all intestinal metaplasia was achieved in 137 (83%). After therapy, patients were followed up for 33 (18–58) months. Among patients who achieved complete elimination of intestinal metaplasia, subsequent recurrent intestinal metaplasia was detected in 48 (35%) and dysplasia in 12 (9%). Among those who only achieved complete elimination of dysplasia, recurrent dysplasia was detected in 6 of 19 (32%). Re-treatment achieved remission in 90% of cases. The current trend is to combine EMR for focal visible lesions with RFA for eradication of remaining Barrett esophagus. Cryotherapy is finding a place for use in salvage therapy. Management should be individualized to use the combinations of therapies to match the unique lesion and patient characteristics. Endoscopic therapy for highly dysplastic Barrett's with HGD and ImCa may be best performed in centers that commit to integrated expertise in interventional endoscopy, radiology, surgery, pathology, and oncology.

PALLIATION OF ESOPHAGEAL CANCER

Most patients with esophageal cancer who present with symptoms and do not have superficial disease are rather diagnosed at an advanced and inoperable stage. These patients often require durable palliation of dysphagia. Although operative palliation can be considered in those without metastatic disease, patients who are poor operative candidates or have locally unresectable disease can achieve palliation of dysphagia with radiation with or without chemotherapy or by endoscopic means. Chemotherapy and radiation can be effective; however; symptom relief may not occur for several weeks and not all patients are candidates for these modalities, such as those with esophageal fistula, poor nutritional status, and weight loss or aspiration.

A variety of endoscopic methods for palliation of malignant dysphagia have been described; however, placement of SEMS provides the most immediate and durable palliation. Endoscopic dilation can provide temporary relief until more definitive treatment can be accomplished; however, this procedure often requires repeat dilation every few weeks, which is not ideal. In addition, there is an associated perforation risk especially in the setting of radiation therapy. Laser therapy fulguration to restore luminal patency has been studied with luminal patency and functional success in 70% to 90% of cases; however, treatments are generally required every other day for a week and relief is often only for several months, at most. Laser therapy is currently rarely performed in the United States. Other therapies such as PDT and APC have been used in small studies[72–75] for palliation, but once again, these have been supplanted by the use of esophageal stents. Results with cryotherapy seem to be promising[76]; however, data supporting its use for palliation of esophageal cancer obstruction are still in its infancy.

Commercially available plastic and metal esophageal expandable stents are in use. The only plastic stent available is called the Polyflex (Boston Scientific, Inc, Natick, MA, USA) made from polyester that is fully covered with silicone. This stent is approved by the US Food and Drug Administration for benign as well as malignant indications. It is intended as a permanent or removable stent. Studies that have compared the Polyflex to traditional partially covered metal stents have noted no difference in palliation; however, stent migration was a substantial issue with the Polyflex stent.[77–79]

Self-Expanding Metal Stents

SEMS are composed of a variety of metal alloys and come in various specifications. While there are nuanced differences in individual stent design, the 3 general themes are fully uncovered, partially covered, and fully covered.

Although covered stents are designed to resist tumor ingrowth, they are associated with higher migration rates, especially if they are fully covered.[80] The covering, however, affords its use in the treatment of fistula or leaks, and they are apt to be readily endoscopically removed. Partially covered stents are uncovered at their ends, which contributes to tissue embedding and anchoring to prevent migration. However, the trade-off is that uncovered or partially covered stents are susceptible to tumor ingrowth and recurrent obstruction.

Most stents are deployed under fluoroscopic and/or endoscopic guidance. Until recently, no available esophageal stent was small enough to pass through the endoscope. The Niti-S stent (Taewoong Medical, Korea) has recently become available as the first through-the-scope esophageal stent. In general, the stenosis should be approximately 6 to 10 mm in diameter to permit passage of the predeployed stent, and therefore prestent delivery dilation may be required. The stenosis should be measured, and a stent length that is approximately 4 cm longer than the tumor or stricture should be chosen. When fluoroscopy is used, the use of external (ie, paper clips secured to patient) or internal markers (frequently hemostatic clips) placed at the margins of the stricture facilitate precise stent positioning. Stent deployment under direct endoscopic visualization is an alternative approach. Once the SEMS is deployed, it expands against the stricture and surrounding tissue and anchors the stent to prevent migration (**Fig. 6**). Patients with large bulky tumors might be evaluated for tracheal compression with CT or bronchoscopy if there is concern for bronchial collapse. SEMS may be successfully placed for the palliation of cervical esophageal malignant obstruction. Care must be taken to position the proximal aspect of the stent just distal or within the upper esophageal sphincter (UES) to allow full closure of the UES. This task may be facilitated by the use of a stent that is deployed from a proximal to distal position (proximal releasing). On the other hand, for distal esophageal tumors, the endoscopist must use caution not to leave an excessive amount of stent below the GE junction within the stomach because the stent can impact on the opposite gastric wall and cause obstruction or ulceration.

SEMS placement is technically successful and highly efficacious in more than 95% of patients with malignant dysphagia,[81,82] allowing patients to tolerate at least full liquids. It is also effective in the management of malignant tracheoesophageal fistula.[83–85]

Numerous types of stents exist and vary in length, shaft diameter, deployment (proximal or distal release systems), and covering extent. The most widely available and commonly used esophageal stents and their characteristics are summarized in **Table 3**.[86] There is not a single study that has compared all the available stents in terms of efficacy, cost, and safety. A meta-analysis that examined 40 randomized trials involving therapies for palliation of esophageal cancer noted that there was no significance in efficacy or complications among the various SEMS.[87] SEMS in comparison to other palliative modalities, however, was quicker in palliating dysphagia.

Subsequent tumor ingrowth and recurrent obstruction after SEMS placement are not uncommon as tumors progress. Therefore, many patients may require additional endoscopic intervention for palliation in 10% to 50% of cases. Durable results can subsequently be achieved by placing a stent within the previously placed stent as treatment of occlusion.

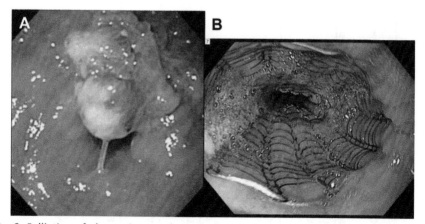

Fig. 6. Palliation of obstructing esophageal adenocarcinoma (A) with SEMS placement (B).

Table 3
Characteristics of available commonly used self-expanding metal esophageal stents

Name	Manufacturer	Composition	Cover Material	Length (Covered Length)	Delivery System Diameter	Unconstrained Diameter
Uncovered						
Ultraflex NG	Boston Scientific	Nitinol	N/A	7 cm 10 cm 15 cm	5 mm	18 mm (proximal flare 23 mm)
Bonastent	EndoChoice	Nitinol	N/A	6 cm 8 cm 10 cm 12 cm 14 cm	6 mm	18-mm (flare 24 mm)
Partially Covered						
Ultraflex	Boston Scientific	Nitinol	Polyurethane	10 cm (7 cm) 12 cm (9 cm) 15 cm (12 cm)	5 mm	18 mm (proximal flare 23 mm) 23 mm (proximal flare 28 mm)
Wallflex	Boston Scientific	Nitinol	Silicone	10 cm (7 cm) 12 cm (9 cm) 15 cm (12 cm)	6.2 mm	18 mm (proximal flare 23 mm) 23 mm (proximal flare 28 mm)
Evolution	Cook Medical	Nitinol	Silicone	8 cm (5 cm) 10 cm (7 cm) 12.5 cm (9.5 cm) 15 cm (12 cm)	8 mm	20 mm
Niti-S	TaeWoong Medical Ltd	Nitinol	Silicone	6 cm (3 cm) 8 cm (5 cm) 10 cm (7 cm) 12 cm (9 cm) 15 cm (12 cm)	5.1–6.5 mm	16 mm (proximal and distal flare 24 mm) 18 mm (proximal and distal flare 26 mm) 20 mm (proximal and distal flare 28 mm)

Fully Covered

Polyflex	Boston Scientific	Polyester	Silicone	9 cm 12 cm 15 cm	12–14 mm	16 mm (proximal flare 20 mm) 18 mm (proximal flare 23 mm) 23 mm (proximal flare 25 mm)
Wallflex	Boston Scientific	Nitinol	Silicone	10 cm 12 cm 15 cm	6.2 mm	18 mm (proximal flare 25 mm; distal flare 23 mm) 23 mm (proximal flare and distal flare 28 mm)
Evolution	Cook Medical	Nitinol	Silicone	8 cm 10 cm 12 cm	8 mm	18 mm (proximal and distal flare 23 mm) 20 mm (proximal and distal flare 25 mm)
ALIMAXX-ES	Merit Endotek (South Jordan, Utah)	Nitinol (laser cut)	Polyurethane	7 cm 10 cm 12 cm	7.4 mm	12 mm (proximal flare 17 mm; distal flare 15 mm) 14 mm (proximal flare 19 mm; distal flare 17 mm) 16 mm (proximal flare 21 mm; distal flare 19 mm) 18 mm (proximal flare 23 mm; distal flare 21 mm) 22 mm (proximal flare 27 mm; distal flare 25 mm)
Niti-S	TaeWoong Medical Ltd	Nitinol	Silicone	6 cm 8 cm 10 cm 12 cm 15 cm	5.8–6.5 mm	16 mm (proximal and distal flare 24 mm) 18 mm (proximal and distal flare 26 mm) 20 mm (proximal and distal flare 28 mm)
Z stent	Cook Medical	Stainless steel	N/A	8 cm 10 cm 12 cm 14 cm	10.3 mm	18 mm (flange 25 mm)

Data from ASGE Technology Committee, Varadarajulu S, Banerjee S, et al. Enteral stents. Gastrointest Endosc 2011;74(3):455–64.

SUMMARY

Advances in endoscopic therapy have resulted in dramatic changes in the way early esophageal cancer is managed as well as in the palliation of dysphagia related to advanced esophageal cancer. EMR and ESD are effective therapies for accurate histopathologic staging and provide a potential for complete cure. Mucosal ablative techniques are effective adjuncts to EMR and ESD and reduce the occurrence of synchronous and metachronous lesions within the Barrett esophagus. The successes of these techniques have made endoscopic therapy the primary means of management of early esophageal cancer. Importantly, it has placed the endoscopist at the multidisciplinary table in discussions of management of esophageal cancer, rather than solely being the diagnostician as in the past. Similarly, SEMS has anchored itself as a durable and immediate modality for the relief of malignant dysphagia from esophageal cancer.

REFERENCES

1. Luna RA, Gilbert E, Hunter JG. High-grade dysplasia and intramucosal adenocarcinoma in Barrett's esophagus: the role of esophagectomy in the era of endoscopic eradication therapy. Curr Opin Gastroenterol 2012;28(4):362–9.
2. Chang AC, Ji H, Birkmeyer NJ, et al. Outcomes after transhiatal and transthoracic esophagectomy for cancer. Ann Thorac Surg 2008;85(2):424–9.
3. Connors RC, Reuben BC, Neumayer LA, et al. Comparing outcomes after transthoracic and transhiatal esophagectomy: a 5-year prospective cohort of 17,395 patients. J Am Coll Surg 2007;205(6):735–40.
4. Hulscher JB, van Sandick JW, de Boer AG, et al. Extended transthoracic resection compared with limited transhiatal resection for adenocarcinoma of the esophagus. N Engl J Med 2002;347(21):1662–9.
5. Omloo JM, Lagarde SM, Hulscher JB, et al. Extended transthoracic resection compared with limited transhiatal resection for adenocarcinoma of the mid/distal esophagus: five-year survival of a randomized clinical trial. Ann Surg 2007; 246(6):992–1000 [discussion: 1000–1].
6. Birkmeyer JD, Siewers AE, Finlayson EV, et al. Hospital volume and surgical mortality in the United States. N Engl J Med 2002;346(15):1128–37.
7. Birkmeyer JD, Stukel TA, Siewers AE, et al. Surgeon volume and operative mortality in the United States. N Engl J Med 2003;349(22):2117–27.
8. Perry KA, Enestvedt CK, Diggs BS, et al. Perioperative outcomes of laparoscopic transhiatal inversion esophagectomy compare favorably with those of combined thoracoscopic-laparoscopic esophagectomy. Surg Endosc 2009; 23(9):2147–54.
9. Perry KA, Enestvedt CK, Pham T, et al. Comparison of laparoscopic inversion esophagectomy and open transhiatal esophagectomy for high-grade dysplasia and stage I esophageal adenocarcinoma. Arch Surg 2009;144(7):679–84.
10. Swanstrom LL, Hansen P. Laparoscopic total esophagectomy. Arch Surg 1997; 132(9):943–7 [discussion: 947–9].
11. Jobe BA, Kim CY, Minjarez RC, et al. Simplifying minimally invasive transhiatal esophagectomy with the inversion approach: lessons learned from the first 20 cases. Arch Surg 2006;141(9):857–65 [discussion: 865–6].
12. Prasad GA, Wu TT, Wigle DA, et al. Endoscopic and surgical treatment of mucosal (T1a) esophageal adenocarcinoma in Barrett's esophagus. Gastroenterology 2009;137(3):815–23.

13. Pech O, Bollschweiler E, Manner H, et al. Comparison between endoscopic and surgical resection of mucosal esophageal adenocarcinoma in Barrett's esophagus at two high-volume centers. Ann Surg 2011;254(1):67–72.

14. Das A, Singh V, Fleischer DE, et al. A comparison of endoscopic treatment and surgery in early esophageal cancer: an analysis of surveillance epidemiology and end results data. Am J Gastroenterol 2008;103(6):1340–5.

15. Pech O, Behrens A, May A, et al. Long-term results and risk factor analysis for recurrence after curative endoscopic therapy in 349 patients with high-grade intraepithelial neoplasia and mucosal adenocarcinoma in Barrett's oesophagus. Gut 2008;57(9):1200–6.

16. Westerterp M, Koppert LB, Buskens CJ, et al. Outcome of surgical treatment for early adenocarcinoma of the esophagus or gastro-esophageal junction. Virchows Arch 2005;446(5):497–504.

17. Ancona E, Rampado S, Cassaro M, et al. Prediction of lymph node status in superficial esophageal carcinoma. Ann Surg Oncol 2008;15(11):3278–88.

18. Barbour AP, Jones M, Brown I, et al. Risk stratification for early esophageal adenocarcinoma: analysis of lymphatic spread and prognostic factors. Ann Surg Oncol 2010;17(9):2494–502.

19. Eguchi T, Nakanishi Y, Shimoda T, et al. Histopathological criteria for additional treatment after endoscopic mucosal resection for esophageal cancer: analysis of 464 surgically resected cases. Mod Pathol 2006;19(3):475–80.

20. Endo M, Yoshino K, Kawano T, et al. Clinicopathologic analysis of lymph node metastasis in surgically resected superficial cancer of the thoracic esophagus. Dis Esophagus 2000;13(2):125–9.

21. Fujita H, Sueyoshi S, Yamana H, et al. Optimum treatment strategy for superficial esophageal cancer: endoscopic mucosal resection versus radical esophagectomy. World J Surg 2001;25(4):424–31.

22. Holscher AH, Bollschweiler E, Schroder W, et al. Prognostic impact of upper, middle, and lower third mucosal or submucosal infiltration in early esophageal cancer. Ann Surg 2011;254(5):802–7 [discussion: 807–8].

23. Leers JM, DeMeester SR, Oezcelik A, et al. The prevalence of lymph node metastases in patients with T1 esophageal adenocarcinoma a retrospective review of esophagectomy specimens. Ann Surg 2011;253(2):271–8.

24. Liu L, Hofstetter WL, Rashid A, et al. Significance of the depth of tumor invasion and lymph node metastasis in superficially invasive (T1) esophageal adenocarcinoma. Am J Surg Pathol 2005;29(8):1079–85.

25. Rice TW, Blackstone EH, Goldblum JR, et al. Superficial adenocarcinoma of the esophagus. J Thorac Cardiovasc Surg 2001;122(6):1077–90.

26. Sepesi B, Watson TJ, Zhou D, et al. Are endoscopic therapies appropriate for superficial submucosal esophageal adenocarcinoma? An analysis of esophagectomy specimens. J Am Coll Surg 2010;210(4):418–27.

27. Shimada H, Nabeya Y, Matsubara H, et al. Prediction of lymph node status in patients with superficial esophageal carcinoma: analysis of 160 surgically resected cancers. Am J Surg 2006;191(2):250–4.

28. Edge SB, Byyrd DR, Compton CC, et al. American Joint Committee on Cancer Staging manual. 7th edition. New York: Springer; 2010. p. 103.

29. van Vliet EP, Eijkemans MJ, Poley JW, et al. Staging of esophageal carcinoma in a low-volume EUS center compared with reported results from high-volume centers. Gastrointest Endosc 2006;63(7):938–47.

30. Bonavina L. Early oesophageal cancer: results of a European multicentre survey. Group Europeen pour l'Etude des Maladies de l'Oesophage. Br J Surg 1995;82(1):98–101.

31. Noguchi H, Naomoto Y, Kondo H, et al. Evaluation of endoscopic mucosal resection for superficial esophageal carcinoma. Surg Laparosc Endosc Percutan Tech 2000;10(6):343–50.
32. Chandawarkar RY, Kakegawa T, Fujita H, et al. Comparative analysis of imaging modalities in the preoperative assessment of nodal metastasis in esophageal cancer. J Surg Oncol 1996;61(3):214–7.
33. Rosch T. Endosonographic staging of esophageal cancer: a review of literature results. Gastrointest Endosc Clin N Am 1995;5(3):537–47.
34. Young PE, Gentry AB, Acosta RD, et al. Endoscopic ultrasound does not accurately stage early adenocarcinoma or high-grade dysplasia of the esophagus. Clin Gastroenterol Hepatol 2010;8(12):1037–41.
35. Thosani N, Singh H, Kapadia A, et al. Diagnostic accuracy of EUS in differentiating mucosal versus submucosal invasion of superficial esophageal cancers: a systematic review and meta-analysis. Gastrointest Endosc 2012;75(2):242–53.
36. Pouw RE, Heldoorn N, Herrero LA, et al. Do we still need EUS in the workup of patients with early esophageal neoplasia? A retrospective analysis of 131 cases. Gastrointest Endosc 2011;73(4):662–8.
37. Ishihara R, Tanaka H, Iishi H, et al. Long-term outcome of esophageal mucosal squamous cell carcinoma without lymphovascular involvement after endoscopic resection. Cancer 2008;112(10):2166–72.
38. ASGE Technology Committee, Kantsevoy SV, Adler DG, et al. Endoscopic mucosal resection and endoscopic submucosal dissection. Gastrointest Endosc 2008;68(1):11–8.
39. Chandrasekhara V, Ginsberg GG. Endoscopic mucosal resection: not your father's polypectomy anymore. Gastroenterology 2011;141(1):42–9.
40. Alvarez Herrero L, Pouw RE, van Vilsteren FG, et al. Safety and efficacy of multiband mucosectomy in 1060 resections in Barrett's esophagus. Endoscopy 2011;43(3):177–83.
41. Pouw RE, van Vilsteren FG, Peters FP, et al. Randomized trial on endoscopic resection-cap versus multiband mucosectomy for piecemeal endoscopic resection of early Barrett's neoplasia. Gastrointest Endosc 2011;74(1):35–43.
42. Yamamoto H. Endoscopic submucosal dissection of early cancers and large flat adenomas. Clin Gastroenterol Hepatol 2005;3(7 Suppl 1):S74–6.
43. Ishihara R, Iishi H, Uedo N, et al. Comparison of EMR and endoscopic submucosal dissection for en bloc resection of early esophageal cancers in Japan. Gastrointest Endosc 2008;68(6):1066–72.
44. Yamaguchi Y, Katusmi N, Aoki K, et al. Resection area of 15 mm as dividing line for choosing strip biopsy or endoscopic submucosal dissection for mucosal gastric neoplasm. J Clin Gastroenterol 2007;41(5):472–6.
45. Fleischer DE, Overholt BF, Sharma VK, et al. Endoscopic radiofrequency ablation for Barrett's esophagus: 5-year outcomes from a prospective multicenter trial. Endoscopy 2010;42(10):781–9.
46. Lyday WD, Corbett FS, Kuperman DA, et al. Radiofrequency ablation of Barrett's esophagus: outcomes of 429 patients from a multicenter community practice registry. Endoscopy 2010;42(4):272–8.
47. Semlitsch T, Jeitler K, Schoefl R, et al. A systematic review of the evidence for radiofrequency ablation for Barrett's esophagus. Surg Endosc 2010;24(12):2935–43.
48. Shaheen NJ, Overholt BF, Sampliner RE, et al. Durability of radiofrequency ablation in Barrett's esophagus with dysplasia. Gastroenterology 2011;141(2):460–8.

49. Hur C, Choi SE, Rubenstein JH, et al. The cost effectiveness of radiofrequency ablation for Barrett's esophagus. Gastroenterology 2012;143(3):567–75.
50. Falk GW. Radiofrequency ablation of Barrett's esophagus: let's not get ahead of ourselves. Dig Dis Sci 2010;55(7):1811–4.
51. Falk GW. Radiofrequency ablation of Barrett's esophagus: should everybody get it? Gastroenterology 2009;136(7):2399–401 [discussion: 2401–2].
52. Titi M, Overhiser A, Ulusarac O, et al. Development of subsquamous high-grade dysplasia and adenocarcinoma after successful radiofrequency ablation of Barrett's esophagus. Gastroenterology 2012;143(3):564–566.e1.
53. Kim HP, Bulsiewicz WJ, Cotton CC, et al. Focal endoscopic mucosal resection before radiofrequency ablation is equally effective and safe compared with radiofrequency ablation alone for the eradication of Barrett's esophagus with advanced neoplasia. Gastrointest Endosc 2012;76(4):733–9.
54. Okoro NI, Tomizawa Y, Dunagan KT, et al. Safety of prior endoscopic mucosal resection in patients receiving radiofrequency ablation of Barrett's esophagus. Clin Gastroenterol Hepatol 2012;10(2):150–4.
55. Gossner L, May A, Stolte M, et al. KTP laser destruction of dysplasia and early cancer in columnar-lined Barrett's esophagus. Gastrointest Endosc 1999;49(1):8–12.
56. Sharma P, Bhattacharyya A, Garewal HS, et al. Durability of new squamous epithelium after endoscopic reversal of Barrett's esophagus. Gastrointest Endosc 1999;50(2):159–64.
57. Yang GR, Zhao LQ, Li SS, et al. Endoscopic Nd: YAG laser therapy in patients with early superficial carcinoma of the esophagus and the gastric cardia. Endoscopy 1994;26(8):681–5.
58. Byrne JP, Armstrong GR, Attwood SE. Restoration of the normal squamous lining in Barrett's esophagus by argon beam plasma coagulation. Am J Gastroenterol 1998;93(10):1810–5.
59. Grade AJ, Shah IA, Medlin SM, et al. The efficacy and safety of argon plasma coagulation therapy in Barrett's esophagus. Gastrointest Endosc 1999;50(1):18–22.
60. Pereira-Lima JC, Busnello JV, Saul C, et al. High power setting argon plasma coagulation for the eradication of Barrett's esophagus. Am J Gastroenterol 2000;95(7):1661–8.
61. Van Laethem JL, Jagodzinski R, Peny MO, et al. Argon plasma coagulation in the treatment of Barrett's high-grade dysplasia and in situ adenocarcinoma. Endoscopy 2001;33(3):257–61.
62. May A, Gossner L, Gunter E, et al. Local treatment of early cancer in short Barrett's esophagus by means of argon plasma coagulation: initial experience. Endoscopy 1999;31(6):497–500.
63. Pech O, Gossner L, May A, et al. Long-term results of photodynamic therapy with 5-aminolevulinic acid for superficial Barrett's cancer and high-grade intraepithelial neoplasia. Gastrointest Endosc 2005;62(1):24–30.
64. Wolfsen HC, Woodward TA, Raimondo M. Photodynamic therapy for dysplastic Barrett esophagus and early esophageal adenocarcinoma. Mayo Clin Proc 2002;77(11):1176–81.
65. Sibille A, Lambert R, Souquet JC, et al. Long-term survival after photodynamic therapy for esophageal cancer. Gastroenterology 1995;108(2):337–44.
66. Pacifico RJ, Wang KK. Role of mucosal ablative therapy in the treatment of the columnar-lined esophagus. Chest Surg Clin N Am 2002;12(1):185–203.
67. Panjehpour M, Overholt BF, Haydek JM, et al. Results of photodynamic therapy for ablation of dysplasia and early cancer in Barrett's esophagus and effect of oral steroids on stricture formation. Am J Gastroenterol 2000;95(9):2177–84.

68. Keeley SB, Pennathur A, Gooding W, et al. Photodynamic therapy with curative intent for Barrett's esophagus with high grade dysplasia and superficial esophageal cancer. Ann Surg Oncol 2007;14(8):2406–10.
69. Greenwald BD, Dumot JA, Abrams JA, et al. Endoscopic spray cryotherapy for esophageal cancer: safety and efficacy. Gastrointest Endosc 2010;71(4):686–93.
70. Halsey KD, Chang JW, Waldt A, et al. Recurrent disease following endoscopic ablation of Barrett's high-grade dysplasia with spray cryotherapy. Endoscopy 2011;43(10):844–8.
71. Guarner-Argente C, Buoncristiano T, Furth EE, et al. Long term outcomes of patients with Barrett's esophagus and high grade dysplasia or early cancer treated with endoluminal therapies with intention to complete eradication. Gastrointest Endosc 2012, in press.
72. McCaughan JS Jr, Ellison EC, Guy JT, et al. Photodynamic therapy for esophageal malignancy: a prospective twelve-year study. Ann Thorac Surg 1996; 62(4):1005–9 [discussion: 1009–10].
73. Lightdale CJ, Heier SK, Marcon NE, et al. Photodynamic therapy with porfimer sodium versus thermal ablation therapy with Nd:YAG laser for palliation of esophageal cancer: a multicenter randomized trial. Gastrointest Endosc 1995;42(6):507–12.
74. Rupinski M, Zagorowicz E, Regula J, et al. Randomized comparison of three palliative regimens including brachytherapy, photodynamic therapy, and APC in patients with malignant dysphagia (CONSORT 1a) (Revised II). Am J Gastroenterol 2011;106(9):1612–20.
75. Eickhoff A, Jakobs R, Schilling D, et al. Prospective nonrandomized comparison of two modes of argon beamer (APC) tumor desobstruction: effectiveness of the new pulsed APC versus forced APC. Endoscopy 2007;39(7):637–42.
76. Cash BD, Johnston LR, Johnston MH. Cryospray ablation (CSA) in the palliative treatment of squamous cell carcinoma of the esophagus. World J Surg Oncol 2007;5:34.
77. Costamagna G, Shah SK, Tringali A, et al. Prospective evaluation of a new self-expanding plastic stent for inoperable esophageal strictures. Surg Endosc 2003;17(6):891–5.
78. Conio M, Repici A, Battaglia G, et al. A randomized prospective comparison of self-expandable plastic stents and partially covered self-expandable metal stents in the palliation of malignant esophageal dysphagia. Am J Gastroenterol 2007; 102(12):2667–77.
79. Verschuur EM, Repici A, Kuipers EJ, et al. New design esophageal stents for the palliation of dysphagia from esophageal or gastric cardia cancer: a randomized trial. Am J Gastroenterol 2008;103(2):304–12.
80. Sharma P, Kozarek R. Practice parameters committee of American College of Gastroenterology. Role of esophageal stents in benign and malignant diseases. Am J Gastroenterol 2010;105(2):258–73 [quiz: 274].
81. Siersema PD, Hop WC, van Blankenstein M, et al. A comparison of 3 types of covered metal stents for the palliation of patients with dysphagia caused by esophagogastric carcinoma: a prospective, randomized study. Gastrointest Endosc 2001;54(2):145–53.
82. Jacobson BC, Hirota W, Baron TH, et al. The role of endoscopy in the assessment and treatment of esophageal cancer. Gastrointest Endosc 2003;57(7):817–22.
83. Chen J, Chen ZM, Pang LW, et al. Deployment of self-expanding metallic stents under fluoroscopic guidance in patients with malignant esophagorespiratory fistula. Hepatogastroenterology 2011;58(105):64–8.

84. Dobrucali A, Caglar E. Palliation of malignant esophageal obstruction and fistulas with self expandable metallic stents. World J Gastroenterol 2010;16(45):5739–45.
85. Talreja JP, Eloubeidi MA, Sauer BG, et al. Fully covered removable nitinol self-expandable metal stents (SEMS) in malignant strictures of the esophagus: a multi-center analysis. Surg Endosc 2012;26(6):1664–9.
86. ASGE Technology Committee, Varadarajulu S, Banerjee S, et al. Enteral stents. Gastrointest Endosc 2011;74(3):455–64.
87. Sreedharan A, Harris K, Crellin A, et al. Interventions for dysphagia in oesophageal cancer. Cochrane Database Syst Rev 2009;(4):CD005048.

Endolumenal Therapies for Gastroesophageal Reflux Disease

Steven Leeds, MD, Kevin Reavis, MD*

KEYWORDS

- Endolumenal • Incisionless fundoplication • Anti-reflux procedure
- Endolumenal plication • Gastroesophageal reflux disease

KEY POINTS

- Patients suffering from gastroesophageal reflux disease that may benefit from endolumenal anti-reflux procedures, which are less invasive than standard surgical approaches.
- The workup for a patient considering an endolumenal anti-reflux procedure is the same as for a patient considering anti-reflux surgery.
- Endolumenal anti-reflux procedures have a similar complication spectrum compared with surgical procedures and are addressed in similar fashion including additional endoscopy or surgical treatment.
- Results from endolumenal anti-reflux procedures are promising however the current therapies are relatively new and require long term data to determine durability.

Gastroesophageal reflux disease (GERD) is a condition that develops as a result of the loss of the anti-reflux barrier created by the lower esophageal sphincter between the stomach and esophagus. The lack of this barrier allows for gastric contents to reflux into the esophagus, causing typical symptoms of heartburn, dysphagia, and regurgitation. If left untreated, GERD may lead to stricture, laryngeal injury, esophagitis, possibly pneumonia, and the development of Barrett's esophagus, which may eventually lead to the development of esophageal adenocarcinoma.[1,2] The prevalence of GERD in Western nations ranges from 10% to 20% in the general population[3,4] and the number of ambulatory visits for GERD in the United States is on the rise.[5]

The medical treatment of GERD is through antisecretory pharmaceuticals such as proton pump inhibitors, histamine$_2$ blockers, and antacids.[6,7] Unfortunately, many patients do not respond to standard dosage regimens, and for those who do, are required to adhere to life-long treatment to avoid recurrent symptoms and progression of disease. Patients who receive little to no symptomatic relief, or who do not wish to use long-term antisecretory medications, can opt for a surgical fundoplication to potentially improve their quality of life. The laparoscopic Nissen fundoplication is the standard surgical treatment for severe GERD with 90% to 94% overall patient

Esophageal and Foregut Surgery, Division of Gastrointestinal and Minimally Invasive Surgery, The Oregon Clinic 4805 Northeast Glisan Street, Suite 6N60, Portland, OR 97213, USA
* Corresponding author.
E-mail address: kreavis@orclinic.com

Gastrointest Endoscopy Clin N Am 23 (2013) 41–51
http://dx.doi.org/10.1016/j.giec.2012.10.010
1052-5157/13/$ – see front matter © 2013 Published by Elsevier Inc.

giendo.theclinics.com

satisfaction and overall outcomes during long-term follow-up.[6,8–13] The main objective of the fundoplication is to restore the anti-reflux barrier by the reconstruction of the lower esophageal sphincter. However, owing to surgical morbidity and common side effects of dysphagia, bloating, flatulence, and difficulty belching and vomiting, patients may be dissuaded from the surgical approach.[14–16]

In search for an alternative and less-invasive approach, attempts to create endolumenal treatments for GERD have been developed and tried over the last couple of decades. Unfortunately, inadequate initial results, failure to objectively treat GERD during long-term follow-up, and overall poor reimbursement, all have contributed to the inability for a single endolumenal treatment to be used for long term.[17] The current endolumenal approaches that are clinically available and will be described are:

1. Transoral incisionless fundoplication (TIF) performed with the EsophyX device (Endogastric Solution Inc, Redmond WA, USA) results in the creation of a 270° to 320° omega-shaped fundoplication.
2. The Stretta procedure (Mederi Therapeutics Inc, Greenwich CT, USA) uses radio-frequency ablation through extended probes into the esophageal musculature to decrease compliance of the lower esophageal sphincter and creates a physiologic anti-reflux barrier.
3. The Endocinch (CR BARD Endoscopic technologies, MA, USA) is used for endolumenal gastroplication. This technology is based on Bard's endoscopic suturing system allowing plication of the gastric fundus from within the lumen to recreate the lower esophageal sphincter, or repair a patulous anti-reflux barrier.[18]

INDICATIONS FOR ENDOLUMENAL TREATMENT FOR GERD

A standard work-up of the GERD patient should be followed whether the patient seeks medical, surgical, or endolumenal treatment. Ideally, patients with objective evidence of moderate to severe GERD without significant hiatal hernia who wish to avoid long-term medical treatment as well as formal laparoscopic or open surgical treatment are candidates for endolumenal treatment. The workup should include the following.

1. *Contrast esophagram*: This evaluates the overall anatomy of the foregut, serves as a preoperative "road map" and identifies hiatal hernias (>2 cm hiatal hernia is a contraindication to current endolumenal treatments).
2. *Upper endoscopy*: This evaluates the esophagogastric mucosa, allows for identification of hiatal hernias and allows for tissue diagnosis of suspect lesions, such as Barrett's esophagus. The histologic results of tissue biopsies can then guide additional treatments.
3. *pH/impedance testing*: The current "gold standard" for the diagnosis of GERD is pH testing. This is necessary to objectively characterize the severity of disease. Impedance testing provides additional value for patients unable to tolerate pH testing while off of antisecretory medication and in those who present with atypical symptoms not adequately characterized with standard pH testing.
4. *High-resolution esophageal manometry*: In any patient with a complaint of dysphagia, manometry is important in characterizing relative esophageal motility and allowing for customization of treatment to avoid overtreating a patient with severe esophageal dysmotility.

Appropriate candidates for endolumenal treatment include those patients with fairly normal anatomy on esophagram, 24-hour pH study results with a Demeester score of at least 14.8 (normal, ≤14.7), no evidence of malignancy on histologic analysis and fairly normal esophageal motility.[19]

Relative contraindications to endolumenal treatment include a body mass index of less than 35 kg/m², Barrett's esophagus, immediate prior esophageal myotomy, esophageal varices, and major connective tissue disorders.

PROCEDURAL TECHNIQUES
TIF

The patient should be prepared for standard upper endoscopy, placing the patient in the left lateral decubitus position. The EsophyX device (**Fig. 1**) and endoscope should be tested on a back table for size compatibility. Next, the patient should have neck extended with bite block with the bed tilted slightly (head higher) to avoid risk of aspiration. General anesthesia with nasotracheal or orotracheal intubation are then induced. Diagnostic upper endoscopy is initially performed to reconfirm no obvious evidence of malignancy or other concerning mucosal abnormalities. Lubrication of the endoscope and EsophyX device with medical grade olive oil or similar lubricant allows for easier manipulation of the component devices. The fastener cartridge and polypropylene H-fasteners are then loaded using the stylet knobs. Next the EsophyX device is placed over the endoscope with the endoscope tip protruding. The EsophyX helical retractor and stylets are locked in retracted position for safety. The EsophyX device and endoscope are introduced as a unit transorally down through the esophagus into the stomach under direct retroflexed visualization. With the EsophyX device facing the greater curvature, the endoscope is withdrawn back to the level of the hinge. The EsophyX device is partially flexed and the endoscope is advanced behind the EsophyX hinge and retroflexed as the EsophyX device is fully flexed into closed position. (Orientation is now as follows: 12 o'clock describes the lesser curvature of the esophagogastric junction; 6 o'clock describes the greater curvature direction located at the Angle of His; 3 o'clock describes the anterior aspect; and 9 o'clock describes the posterior aspect; **Fig. 2**). The helical retractor is advanced into the 12 o'clock position and tissue is secured. The tissue mold is partially opened at the 6 o'clock position and closed over 2 to 3 cm of tissue. The invaginator is then engaged. The tissue mold is swung toward 1 o'clock and gastric disinflation is simultaneously performed. Gastric insufflation is followed by advancement of anterior and posterior stylets and fasteners (via the fastener pushers) in sequential fashion (**Fig. 3**). The tissue mold is unlocked, repositioned, and relocked. Two more fasteners are deployed. The tissue invaginator is released. The tissue mold is swung around the 12 o'clock position and similar maneuvers are used to place a total of 4 fasteners at the 11 o'clock position. The helical retractor is released and re-engaged at the 6 o'clock position. The tissue invaginator is re-engaged. Two fasteners are deployed after grasping 3 cm of tissue in the tissue mold at the 8 o'clock position and then at the 4 o'clock position. There is no need for tissue swinging or disinflation during these fastener deployments.

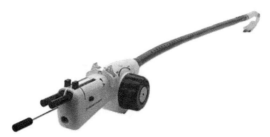

Fig. 1. EsophyX device. (*Courtesy of* Endogastric Solutions, Inc. Redwood City, CA, USA; with permission.)

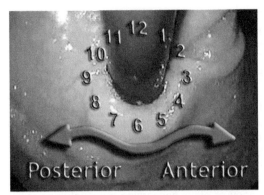

Fig. 2. Clockface orientation of retroflexed view of gastroesophageal junction. (*Courtesy of* Endogastric Solutions, Inc. Redwood City, CA, USA; with permission.)

A total of 12 fasteners are deployed approximately 1 to 2 cm above the esophageal Z-line. Additional fasteners can be deployed as necessary to develop a 2 to 3 cm 270° to 320° omega shaped esophagogastric wrap.

The endoscope and EsophyX device (with stylets and helical retractor locked in retracted position) are then removed. Before concluding the procedure, a final upper endoscopy is performed to confirm that an adequate fundoplication has been created and that no perforation or bleeding is present. The patient is extubated and taken to the recovery room, before going to the ward or home for postoperative care.

Stretta

Begin by preparing the patient for standard upper endoscopy, placing the patient in the left lateral decubitus position.[20] The patient should have neck extended with a bite block in place then tilt the bed slightly (head higher) to avoid risk of aspiration. Prepare the patient using standard technique for monopolar electrosurgery by initially applying the return electrode pad to a cleaned and hairless area on the patient's right mid scapular area off the mid line. The recommended treatments for Stretta are 4 antegrade treatment levels in and around the lower esophageal sphincter, 5 mm apart from

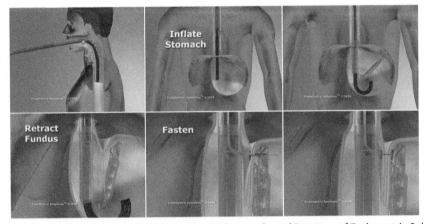

Fig. 3. Transoral incisionless fundoplication (TIF) procedure. (*Courtesy of* Endogastric Solutions, Inc. Redwood City, CA, USA; with permission.)

each other (two 1-minute treatment sites per level at home position and the 45° to right for treatment levels 1 to 4) and 2 pull-back treatment levels in the gastric cardia (three 1-minute treatment sites per level, home position, 30° to the left and 30° to the right of home for levels 5 and 6). Endoscopic inspection of the esophagus, measurement of distance from Z-line to bite block confirms the location and depth of the patients Z-line (squamocolumnar tissue) versus the fixed oral bite block. The Z-line serves as the reference landmark for the first 4 (antegrade) of 6 total treatment levels. A guide wire is then passed through the scope and into the stomach of the patient to run the Stretta Catheter over. From Standby mode, push the Power On/Mode button to advance to Ready mode, the catheter is lubricated (**Fig. 4**) and inserted into the esophagus down to the Z-line measurement and then retracted to a position 1 cm above the Z-line for treatment level 1. Placement is confirmed versus the bite block. Next suction is attached to the catheter. The pressure release valve is attached to the air syringe. Thirty milliliters of air are drawn into the syringe and inserted into the insufflation port on the Stretta Catheter until the pressure release valve releases excess air. Once the balloon is inflated, extend the needles that go into the tissue of the esophagus.

Antegrade treatments
The needles are extended to the full extent, and then retracted to the treatment depth (**Fig. 5**). Impedance readings are monitored on the generator screen. Optimal impedance readings below 200 indicate proper placement of needles. Once proper placement is confirmed the foot pedal is depressed once, beginning a 1-minute treatment cycle. Once the 1-minute cycle is complete the generator will go into a "pause" mode to allow for repositioning of the catheter.

Between treatments
Retract the needles and deflate the balloon. Pull the catheter back up to 25 cm to allow for suction, rotate 45° to the right and then advance the catheter down the guide wire to desired depth as measured against the bite block. If resistance is experienced while pulling the catheter back, release suction, and then reestablish suction before next treatment. (Note: Use the shaft of the catheter as well as the handle to rotate, not just the handle). Reinflate balloon using the pressure release valve to prevent overinflation. The foot pedal is depressed to begin the next 1-minute treatment cycle and a second set of lesions is created, establishing the first antegrade ring of 8 lesions. Three more rings are created in this manner: 0.5 cm above the Z-line, at the Z-line, and 0.5 cm below the Z-line.

Cardia pull-back/retrograde treatments
For these treatment levels, do not pull back higher than 2 cm above the Z-line, and do not advance into the stomach lower than 2 cm below the Z-line. For treatment level 5, advance the catheter into the fundus of the stomach and inflate the balloon with 25 mL

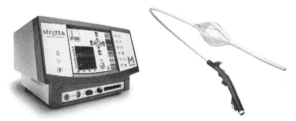

Fig. 4. Stretta device and control box. (*Courtesy of* Mederi Therapeutics Inc., Greenwich, CT, USA; with permission. © 2012 Mederi Therapeutics Inc.)

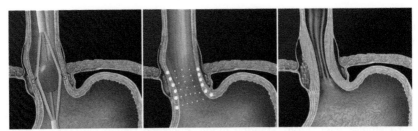

Fig. 5. Stretta procedure. (*Courtesy of* Mederi Therapeutics Inc., Greenwich, CT, USA; with permission. © 2012 Mederi Therapeutics Inc.)

of air, slowly pull back the inflated balloon against the hiatus until snug. Extend the needles and deliver the first of three 1-minute treatments at this level. At the completion of the first one-minute treatment cycle, retract the needles, advance into the stomach, rotate 30° to the right, pull back until snug and extend needles and repeat. For the third treatment on this level, rotate catheter 30° to the left of first treatment. For treatment level 6, retract needles and advance the catheter again into the fundus of the stomach. Deflate balloon and then reinflate with 22 mL, then pull back against the hiatus to fit snugly, above treatment level 5. Extend the needles and deliver the first treatment cycle in this level. After the first treatment cycle, retract the needles, advance into the stomach, rotate 30° to the right, extend needles and repeat, then repeat cycle again 30° to the left of first treatment. After completion of 6 levels of treatment, the balloon is deflated and the catheter is removed. An endoscopic inspection of the treatment area should confirm safe delivery and completion of Stretta Therapy. The patient is awakened or extubated depending on anesthesia used and taken to the recovery room, before going to the ward or home for postoperative care.

Endocinch

Once again the patient should be prepared for standard upper endoscopy, placing the patient in the left lateral decubitus position. The neck should be extended with bite block and the bed tilted slightly (head higher) to avoid risk of aspiration. General anesthesia is next induced with nasotracheal or orotracheal intubation. Diagnostic upper endoscopy is initially performed to reconfirm no obvious evidence of malignancy or other concerning mucosal abnormalities. With the Endocinch attached to the endoscope, it should be passed under direct visualization to the Z-line. The scope should be passed just beyond the Z-line and the suction activated to pull the mucosa to the suction port at the end of the scope (**Fig. 6**). The preloaded suture should be deployed at that point to pass the suture through the mucosa. Continue the same process to create the desired suture configuration (ie, figure of 8). Then, cinch the suture tight with the Endocinch and cut the suture to create the knot approximating the mucosa. This should be repeated around the gastric cardia to create the desired anti-reflux barrier.

FOLLOW-UP AFTER ENDOLUMENAL THERAPY

A liquid diet is commonly prescribed immediately after endolumenal treatments and advanced to regular food as the patient tolerates. Assertive anti-nausea medication is also helpful to avoid stress to the treated area.

Standard post anti-reflux surgery follow-up clinic appointments are appropriate with additional evaluations such as upper endoscopy and/or pH testing being instituted if patients report recurrent symptoms.

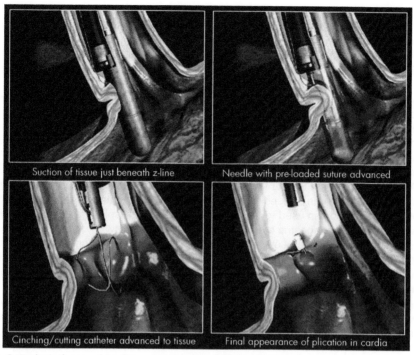

Suction of tissue just beneath z-line

Needle with pre-loaded suture advanced

Cinching/cutting catheter advanced to tissue

Final appearance of plication in cardia

Fig. 6. Endocinch procedure. (*From* Arts J, Tack J, Galmiche JP. Endoscopic antireflux procedures. Gut 2004;53(8):1207–14. *Courtesy of* Bard, Inc. Murray Hill, NJ.)

RESULTS

TIF has been shown by Cadiere and colleagues[21–24] to be safe and effective in humans at 12 months with reports of 85% discontinuation of proton pump inhibitors and 75% elimination of GERD-related symptoms. Three-year follow-up data from Belgium and The Netherlands as well as 2-year follow-up data from Italy have revealed promising longer term results regarding symptom control with around 70% of patients not needing antisecretory medication after TIF. Preprocedural esophageal motility disorders and hiatal hernia were associated with early recurrence of GERD symptoms.[25–27] Patients with these specific conditions should be counseled regarding alternative surgical approaches to increase the likelihood of an optimal outcome.

TIF has been used in the United States since 2007 for treatment of moderate to severe GERD. One advantage of TIF over surgical treatment is the application of this procedure in patients who have undergone prior gastric operations, including surgical fundoplication as well as antrectomy (as part of a pancreaticoduodenectomy).[28,29] This subset of patients offers a potentially hostile environment for standard laparoscopic and open approaches, but a straightforward approach for endolumenal treatments. Several case series have been reported from academic university and community centers in the United States with results ranging from dissatisfaction and overt failure in nearly half of patients early on to more recent objective successful treatment and high level satisfaction in a majority of patients.[30–33] Currently, the Randomized EsophyX versus Sham/Placebo Controlled TIF Trial: The RESPECT Study (Clinical Trials.gov NCT01136980) is being conducted. This is a multicenter, randomized, controlled trial in the United States proposed to objectively determine the effectiveness of TIF during a 6-month follow-up period. In addition to this the

TIF versus Medical Proton Pump Inhibitor Management of Refractory GERD Symptoms (TEMPO) trial (Clinical Trials.gov NCT01647958) is a second multicenter, randomized, controlled trial underway that seeks to evaluate the effectiveness of TIF over a 6-month period in controlling GERD symptoms.

Stretta has a relatively long track record of successful clinical outcomes with more than 1400 patients analyzed in over 20 studies. Owing to financial considerations, the Stretta technology was largely unavailable between 2006 and 2008 yet has returned and is now clinically available. Studies have shown it to be effective not only in reducing symptoms of GERD and improving quality of life scores, but objective reduction in esophageal acid exposure and improvements in esophagogastric physiology have also been demonstrated during more than 12 months of follow-up (Melvin WS, personal communication, 2010).

An advantage of the Stretta technology is its design. Because it has no retracting component, Stretta can be used in challenging anatomic situations; it requires minimal working space and can used to treat the lower esophageal sphincter of patients who have undergone prior gastric bypass or subtotal gastrectomy.

Endocinch therapy has been shown to provide good results in long-term follow-up in the past. The endolumenal gastroplication using Endocinch significantly reduces the occurrence of GERD symptoms, use of GERD medications, and the cost of maintenance drug regimens. These outcomes were supported with objective data in 24-hour pH monitoring. Despite these early results, the data are still limited. However, there are new data that come from Japan showing that about 60% of patients benefit from endolumenal gastroplication with Endocinch with regard to GERD symptoms at 24 months.[34] It has also been shown to be safe and effective in the pediatric population.[35] This provides a great way for surgeons to suture within the gastrointestinal tract without the need for surgery through laparoscopy or laparotomy.

COMPLICATIONS

Perforation is the most serious intraprocedural complication feared. The common causes and sources of prevention are as follows. Overassertiveness while placing either the EsophyX device or Stretta device can result in esophageal injury. This can be prevented by recognizing resistant anatomy despite optimized patient positioning and deferring to medical treatment or formal surgical anti-reflux treatment. Too aggressive suturing with the Endocinch can result in full-thickness passage of the suture. These suture passes may result in perforations if the tissue tears or becomes ischemic resulting in breakdown. Care with partial thickness suture passes, and recognition of friable tissue can avoid this. Recognition and management are key. Mucosal injury requires only close observation. Transmural injury requires definitive source control through either laparoscopy/laparotomy or thoracoscopy/thoracotomy or cervical repair of the injured esophageal or gastric segment. Endolumenal stenting of esophageal injuries is a technique under current investigation; however, the appropriate application of this technology is yet to be formalized.

Endolumenal bleeding after TIF, Stretta, or Endocinch is caused by penetration of submucosal vessels. The avoidance of attempting to treat patients with esophageal varices is imperative. Suture passes with the Endocinch that result in mucosa only have the propensity to tear and cause mucosal bleeding. Endolumenal bleeding after TIF can be controlled with direct pressure of the clasped tissue mold for a period of a minute or more. Ongoing bleeding after this maneuver or bleeding after Stretta or Endocinch can usually be controlled through standard endolumenal methods with injection/cautery or via the placement of clips.

Mediastinal/abdominal abscess can result from penetration of the left crus during TIF or assertive movements with the extended Stretta probes via eventual microperforation of the esophagogastric fundoplication or lower esophageal sphincter respectively. Recognizing the left crus, applying the tissue invaginator to advance the esophagus during TIF and placement of fasteners to the abdominal portion of the esophagus will help to prevent this complication. Abscess should be suspected in patients displaying signs of thoracic infection in the post procedure period. Radiographic studies provide confirmation. Source control with percutaneous abdominal or thoracic drainage along with indicated antimicrobial treatment is usually adequate.

Recurrent symptoms have been noted after technical error, misdiagnosis or stress to the operative field. Adequate training and technique, thorough objective work-up to confirm the diagnosis and assertive anti-nausea therapy during the post procedure period reduces the likelihood of recurrent symptoms. Objective evaluation as performed in the pre-procedure period is warranted to confirm recurrent disease. Re-performing the treatment in appropriate patients is possible with TIF, Stretta or Endocinch technologies.

FUTURE DIRECTIONS

TIF Stretta and Endocinch all seem technically safe in well-selected patients, including those with prior esophageal and gastric surgeries. Long-term effectiveness with regard to these technologies is being evaluated with ongoing investigations. Given the current enthusiasm for increasingly less invasive surgical techniques, the inertia for endolumenal therapies continues to grow. In addition to the 3 techniques discussed in this article, other endolumenal therapies for GERD have initiated trials in Europe and the United States. These pursue similar fundoplication or lower esophageal sphincter reconstruction using simpler techniques with fewer steps. One in particular combines a surgical stapler, ultrasound guidance and a miniature video camera on the tip of a flexible endoscope to create an anterior gastroesophageal fundoplication and is also currently involved in a multicenter clinical trial.[36] Because all endolumenal approaches to GERD evolve, objective evaluation for symptom resolution and reduced esophageal acid exposure with improved esophagogastric physiology remain a constant.

REFERENCES

1. Group Health Cooperative. Clinical review criteria CR BARD's endoscopic suturing system (endocinch therapy, endoluminal plication) for the treatment of GERD. Seattle, Wa: Group Health Cooperative; 2010.
2. Fock KM, Poh CH. Gastroesophageal reflux disease. J Gastroenterol 2010;45: 808–15.
3. Dent J, El-Serag HB, Wallander MA, et al. Epidemiology of gastroesophageal reflux disease: a systematic review. Gut 2005;54:710–7.
4. Locke GR III, Talley NJ, Fett SL, et al. Prevalence and clinical spectrum of gastroesophageal reflux: a population-based study in Olmsted County, Minnesota. Gastroenterology 1997;112:1448–56.
5. Friedenberg FK, Hanlon A, Vanar V, et al. Trends in gastroesophageal reflux disease as measured by the National Ambulatory Medical Care Survey. Dig Dis Sci 2010;55:1911–7.
6. Allgood PC, Bachmann M. Medical or surgical treatment for chronic gastroesophageal reflux? A systematic review of published evidence of effectiveness. Eur J Surg 2000;166:713–21.

7. Dent J. Landmarks in the understanding and treatment of reflux disease. J Gastroenterol Hepatol 2009;24(Suppl 3):S5–14.
8. Dallemagne B, Weerts J, Markiewicz S, et al. Clinical results of laparoscopic fundoplication at ten years after surgery. Surg Endosc 2006;20:159–65.
9. Lafullarde T, Watson DI, Jamieson GG, et al. Laparoscopic Nissen fundoplication: five-year results and beyond. Arch Surg 2001;136:180–4.
10. Hunter JG, Trus TL, Branum GD, et al. A physiologic approach to laparoscopic fundoplication for gastroesophageal reflux disease. Ann Surg 1996;223:673–87.
11. Lundell L, Miettinen P, Myrvold HE, et al. Seven-year follow-up of a randomized clinical trial comparing proton-pump inhibition with surgical therapy for reflux oesophagitis. Br J Surg 2007;94:198–203.
12. Mahon D, Rhodes M, Decadt B, et al. Randomized clinical trial of laparoscopic Nissen fundoplication compared with proton-pump inhibitors for treatment of chronic gastroesophageal reflux. Br J Surg 2005;92:695–9.
13. Terry M, Smith CD, Branum GD, et al. Outcomes of laparoscopic fundoplication for gastroesophageal reflux disease and paraesophageal hernia. Surg Endosc 2001;15:691–9.
14. Coelho JC, Wiederkehr JC, Campos AC, et al. Conversions and complications of laparoscopic treatment of gastroesophageal reflux disease. J Am Coll Surg 1999;189:356–61.
15. Kamolz T, Granderath FA, Bammer T, et al. Dysphagia and quality of life after laparoscopic Nissen fundoplication in patients with and without prosthetic reinforcement of the hiatal crura. Surg Endosc 2002;16:572–7.
16. Lundell L. Complications after anti-reflux surgery. Best Pract Res Clin Gastroenterol 2004;18:935–45.
17. Reavis KM, Nguyen AK, editors. Endolumenal approaches to gastroesophageal disease. The SAGES manual. New York: Springer; 2012. p. 247–60.
18. Introduction of BARD EndocinchTM Suturing System. Available at: http://www.touchbriefings.com/pdf/790/bard.pdf. Accessed August 10, 2012.
19. Demeester TR, Johnson LF, Joseph GJ, et al. Patterns of gastroesophageal reflux in health and disease. Ann Surg 1976;184:459–70.
20. Mederi Therapeutics Inc. Instructions for use. 2011.
21. Cadiere GB, Buset M, Muls V, et al. Antireflux transoral incisionless fundoplication using EsophyX: 12-month results of a prospective multicenter study. World J Surg 2008;32:1676–88.
22. Cadiere GB, Rajan A, Germay O, et al. Endolumenal fundoplication by a transoral device for the treatment of GERD: a feasibility study. Surg Endosc 2008;22:333–42.
23. Hoppo T, Immanuel A, Shuchert M, et al. Transoral incisionless fundoplication 2.0 procedure using esophyX for gastroesophageal reflux disease. J Gastrointest Surg 2010;14(12):1895–901.
24. Hays RD, Sherbourne CD, Mazel RM. The RAND 36-item health survey 1.0. Health Econ 1993;2:217–27.
25. Muls V, Eckardt AJ, Marchese M, et al. Three-year results of a multicenter prospective study of transoral incisionless fundoplication. Surg Innov 2012 Sep 11. [Epub ahead of print].
26. Witteman BP, Strijkers R, de Vries E, et al. Transoral incisionless fundoplication for treatment of gastroesophageal reflux disease in clinical practice. Surg Endosc 2012;26:3307–15.
27. Testoni PA, Vailati C, Testoni S, et al. Transoral incisionless fundoplication (TIF 2.0) with EsophyX for gastroesophageal reflux disease: long-term results and findings affecting outcome. Surg Endosc 2012;26(5):1425–35.

28. Ginsberg GG, Barkun AN, Bosco JJ, et al. Technology Status Report: Endoscopic Anti-Reflux Procedures. 2002;56(5):625–8.
29. Nguyen A, Vo T, Nguyen X, et al. Transoral incisionless fundoplication: initial experience in patients referred to an integrated academic institution. Am Surg 2011;77(10):1386–9.
30. Bergman S, Mikami DJ, Hazey JW, et al. Endoluminal fundoplication with EsophyX: the initial North American experience. Surg Innov 2008;15:166–70.
31. Cadiere GB, Van Sante N, Graves JE, et al. Two-year results of a feasibility study on antireflux – using EsophyX. Surg Endosc 2009;23:957–64.
32. Demyttenaere SV, Bergman S, Pham T, et al. Transoral incisionless fundoplication for gastroesophageal reflux disease in an unselected patient population. Surg Endosc 2010;24:854–8.
33. Bell RC, Freeman KD. Clinical and pH-metric outcomes of transoral esophago-gastric fundoplication for the treatment of gastroesophageal reflux disease. Surg Endosc 2011;25(6):1975–84.
34. Ozawa S, Kumai K, Higuchi K, et al. Short-term and long-term outcome of endo-luminal gastroplication for the treatment of GERD: the first multicenter trial in Japan. J Gastroenterol 2009;44(7):675–84.
35. Thomson M, Antao B, Hall S, et al. Medium-term outcome of endoluminal gastro-plication with the EndoCinch device in children. J Pediatr Gastroenterol Nutr 2008;46(2):172–7.
36. Medigus SRS Endoscope. Available at: http://www.medigus.com/. Accessed August 10, 2012.

Achalasia

Stavros N. Stavropoulos, MD[a,b,*], Rani Modayil, MD[a],
David Friedel, MD[a,c]

KEYWORDS

- Achalasia • Peroral endoscopic myotomy • Endoluminal treatment
- Endoscopic submucosal dissection • Natural orifice transluminal endoscopic surgery

KEY POINTS

- POEM clearly is a paradigm shift in achalasia therapy.
- With POEM, essentially an endoscopic procedure with its associated convenience and less invasiveness can duplicate clinical results of a time-tested surgical procedure (LHM).
- Further refinements of the POEM technique are expected.

INTRODUCTION AND SCOPE OF THE PROBLEM

Achalasia is an uncommon esophageal motility disorder where the lower esophageal sphincter (LES) fails to relax in response to swallowing. The term is derived from Greek (α = non, $\chi\alpha\lambda\alpha\sigma\iota\alpha$ = relaxation). Achalasia is characterized by dysphagia and, on occasion, chest pain, regurgitation, aspiration pneumonia, and weight loss.[1] Esophageal manometry reveals aperistalsis confined to the distal two-thirds of the esophagus and abnormal LES relaxation, although the diagnosis is often suggested by an esophageal contrast study demonstrating characteristic distal "bird's beak" esophageal narrowing. Endoscopic and surgical therapy is focused on LES disruption rather than the motility abnormalities in the rest of the esophagus. Achalasia has no epidemiologic predilection for any demographic group, affects men and women equally, and may occur at any age.[2] It has an incidence of approximately 1 per 200,000 and a prevalence of approximately 1 per 10,000.[2] Selective loss of the inhibitory neurons in the myenteric plexus causes unopposed excitation of the LES.[3] No current therapy is considered curative for life. Dysphagia relief is the main treatment objective. With progressive deterioration of esophageal function, the natural evolution of achalasia leads to end-stage sigmoid megaesophagus that may eventually require an esophagectomy in at least 5% of patients.[4]

[a] Division of Gastroenterology, Hepatology and Nutrition, Winthrop University Hospital, 222 Station Plaza North, Suite 429, Mineola, NY 11501, USA; [b] Department of Medicine, College of Physicians and Surgeons, Columbia University, 630 West 168th Street, New York, NY 10032-3784, USA; [c] Department of Medicine, SUNY Stony Brook University School of Medicine, 101 Nicholls Road, Stony Brook, NY 11794, USA
* Corresponding author.
E-mail address: sstavropoulos@winthrop.org

Gastrointest Endoscopy Clin N Am 23 (2013) 53–75
http://dx.doi.org/10.1016/j.giec.2012.10.008
1052-5157/13/$ – see front matter © 2013 Elsevier Inc. All rights reserved.

PAST MANAGEMENT OPTIONS

More than 20 studies have validated the efficacy of pneumatic dilation (PD).[5] Long-term efficacy may exceed 90% but usually requires serial dilations.[6–8] Thus, PD can yield excellent results in experienced hands if patients are monitored for recurrent symptoms. The risk of PD perforation ranges to 8%.[9] There are no well-validated risk factors for PD perforation.[10] PD is more likely to be successful in older patients with dysphagia (and little chest pain) and a compatible high-resolution manometry.[11] A pivotal randomized controlled trial (RCT) by Boeckxstaens and colleagues[12] compared PD with laparoscopic Heller myotomy (LHM). There was little difference between the groups at 1 year in terms of dysphagia and other symptoms, and at 2 years there was no significant difference in terms of LES pressure, esophageal emptying, or quality of life. However, in the United States, LHM remains the undisputed first-line treatment for achalasia because of a well-validated, durable clinical response and medicolegal concerns regarding perforation with PD. Pasricha and coworkers[13,14] introduced the concept of Botox injection (BTI) for achalasia in 1995 and their subsequent prospective study demonstrated a symptomatic response in two-thirds of patients with a mean follow-up of 2.4 years. They found a better response in those with moderate LES pressures, older subjects, and in those with "vigorous" achalasia. Response rates in other studies averaged 78% at 1 month but fell to 49% at 1 year.[7] Repeat injections modestly increase efficacy.[15] The consensus is that BTI yields inferior clinical response in achalasia compared with PD and myotomy.[16] The safety profile for BTI is excellent. This aspect and the ease of technique may account for the continued popularity of BTI despite its inferior efficacy. It is a viable option for the frail elderly and others who could not tolerate perforation and surgery.[17]

Recent investigational endoluminal treatments include ethanolamine injection in the LES[18] and use of self-expanding metal stents. Small pilot studies in the United States and Europe yielded poor results with self-expanding metal stents with significant complications.[19,20] However, a study using covered 30-mm self-expanding metal stents from a single center in China[21] demonstrated the safety of deploying a 30-mm self-expanding metal stent in 75 achalasia patients with no perforations or 30-day mortality.[22] The 100% clinical remission rate is puzzling because the stents were removed within 5 days. A prospective study comparing 30-mm self-expanding metal stent insertion in achalasia versus 30-mm PD demonstrated comparable if not superior clinical results in the stent group.[23] These stents were specially designed for achalasia dilation (**Fig. 1**). The 30-mm self-expanding metal stent seems to be optimal in terms of efficacy and lower risk of migration than smaller stents.[24] However, Dua[25] urges caution in using self-expanding metal stents for benign esophageal disease including achalasia.

PERORAL ENDOSCOPIC MYOTOMY

In 2007, Sumiyama and coworkers reported a technique of transluminal access via a submucosal tunnel approach which offsets the mucosotomy and myotomy sites and thus allows rapid secure closure with clips placed at the mucosotomy site.[26] This technique was utilized in a survival animal study by Pasricha and colleagues to perform endoscopic LES myotomy.[27] Shortly thereafter, Inoue and coworkers[28] used this technique to perform endoscopic LES myotomy in a patient with achalasia and coined the elegant acronym POEM (peroral endoscopic myotomy). In 2009, at Winthrop University Hospital, the authors' team was the second in the world to perform POEM[29] initiating the first prospective institutional review board–approved

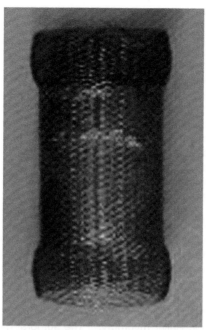

Fig. 1. Self-expanding metallic stent for achalasia. (*Courtesy of* Cheng YS, Ma F, Li YD, et al. Temporary self-expanding metallic stents for achalasia: a prospective study with a long-term follow-up. World J Gastroenterol 2010;16(40):5111–7; with permission.)

trial outside of Japan. Over the past 3 years only about 20 centers around the world (nine in the United States) have established POEM programs but the number is now expanding exponentially as preliminary data from early adopters have demonstrated excellent safety and efficacy. Because of this exponential growth, the scant peer-reviewed publications lag well behind the rapidly expanding experience with POEM. Therefore, this article depends more than is customary on data that have not yet been published in full form. These include data from the authors' POEM series, likely the largest series with longest follow-up in the United States, and a comprehensive international POEM survey (IPOEMS) that was recently completed in July of 2012 (unpublished data). Unfortunately, only very limited subsets of these data are presented here because they will be appearing in full in upcoming dedicated, peer-reviewed publications. The series currently includes a total of 43 patients that underwent POEM. The data on the first 29 patients that have reached minimum follow-up of more than 3 months (range, 3–34 months) were presented at Digestive Disease Week 2012.[30] IPOEMS was performed by Stavropoulos and Savides as part of the annual Natural Orifice Surgery Consortium for Assessment and Research NOTES summit meeting in July 2012. It was motivated by the need to obtain additional data to supplement the scant literature to be used in composing an upcoming Natural Orifice Surgery Consortium for Assessment and Research white paper on POEM. A total of 16 participating centers (five in Asia, four in Europe, and seven in the United States) with a combined POEM volume of 841 POEMS, including all centers around the world with POEM volumes of greater than 30 procedures, provided comprehensive detailed data on every aspect of POEM, including training, technique, periprocedural management, efficacy, complications, and future directions.

INDICATIONS AND CONTRAINDICATIONS

IPOEMS data reveal that some centers have expanded POEM indications beyond typical nonspastic achalasia (Chicago classification I, II), which accounted for only 72.4% of the 841 cases with the remainder performed for, in decreasing frequency, nutcracker, hypertensive LES, spastic achalasia (type III) and diffuse esophageal spasm (**Table 1**). A longer myotomy is advocated for spastic motility disorders with long spastic distal esophageal segments. This can be easier to perform by POEM than LHM and may account for the surprisingly rapid expansion of POEM indications to include such disorders in one-quarter of cases. A case report on use of POEM in diffuse esophageal spasm reported a myotomy length of 17 cm, much longer than the 8 to 10 cm length usually achievable by LHM.[31]

POEM has been extensively applied in patients with prior failed PD and BTI. Among the five published series, four reported substantial numbers of patients undergoing POEM after prior BTI or PD ranging from 18% to 80% (**Table 2**), but none of the investigators performed a formal subgroup analysis. Based on experience with POEM after PD and BTI, it seems that, as in the LHM literature, prior BTI is more problematic than PD. The statement from von Renteln and coworkers[36] that POEM in previously treated patients is "more challenging but feasible" seems to capture the majority view.

POEM after failed LHM presents special challenges because of scar formation and frequent presence of fundoplication. Inoue and coworkers[39] reported successful POEM on seven patients after failed LHM and the Shanghai group in six patients after prior failed thoracoscopic Heller myotomy.[40] The authors, having successfully performed POEM in a patient with failed prior Heller myotomy as the thirty-seventh patient in their series, agree with the recommendation by Inoue and Zhou for minimum POEM operator volume of at least 30 cases before tackling failed LHM cases.

Based on the LHM literature, patients with severe sigmoidization and megaesophagus (end-stage achalasia) respond poorly to LHM and, even though myotomy can be considered initially as a less invasive approach, many patients may ultimately come to esophagectomy.[41] Based on the similarities between POEM and LHM one could anticipate similarly limited efficacy of POEM in end-stage achalasia. Inoue and

Table 1
POEM indications and contraindications

Standard Indications	Possible Extended Indications[a]	Contraindications
Achalasia	Spastic motility disorders other than achalasia (diffuse esophageal spasm, hypertensive LES, nutcracker esophagus)	Severe pulmonary disease
Prior failed treatment with botulinum toxin injection and pneumatic dilation		Severe coagulopathy
		Extensive esophageal mucosal ablation (radiofrequency ablation, EMR, ESD)
	Failed Heller myotomy	Esophageal or chest irradiation
	Age extremes (children, very elderly >80 y old)	
	End-stage achalasia (severe sigmoidization, megaesophagus)	
	Comorbid conditions other than those listed under "contraindications"	

[a] Additional data required regarding safety and efficacy.

coworkers[32] reported successful POEM in 17 patients that included 11 of 17 grade II (3.5–6 cm) and 3 of 17 grade III (>6 cm) patients without, however, specific subgroup analysis. They reported POEM in 5 of 17 patients with moderate (S1) sigmoid esophagus with good efficacy but a lower decrease in the LES pressure compared with the 12 patients without sigmoid esophagus.[32] Inoue and coworkers[39] reported successful POEM in 16 of 105 patients with sigmoid achalasia. The authors and others have not excluded end-stage patients a priori from POEM consideration (they have successfully performed POEM in patients with severe sigmoidization and esophageal dilation as extreme as 11.5 cm). Therefore, data regarding the technical challenge and possible diminished efficacy of POEM in these patients should be forthcoming.

POEM has been reported in children as young as 3[37] and 6,[38] again without subgroup analysis. Minimal data are available on patients older than 80 years old. Thirteen percent of the authors' series involved patients older than 80 (81–93) who, despite significant comorbidities, had excellent POEM efficacy and safety.

With regards to comorbid conditions, literature data are essentially nonexistent. Useful data were extracted from the IPOEMS survey. Participants were asked to comment whether POEM was contraindicated in 17 clinical scenarios including morbid obesity, cardiac, pulmonary, renal, hepatic, immune system, and clotting system comorbidities of various severities, prior mediastinal surgery, and interventions causing esophageal submucosal fibrosis (esophageal mucosal ablation/endoscopic mucosal resection (EMR)/endoscopic submucosal dissection (ESD), esophageal or chest radiation). The only comorbidities for which there was substantial consensus that they constitute contraindications to POEM were severe pulmonary disease, significant coagulopathy, esophageal mucosal ablation/EMR/ESD, and esophageal or chest radiation.

PROCEDURE
Preparation

Full liquid diet is instituted for 1 to 5 days (center dependent) and nothing by mouth for 8 to 24 hours. Some centers perform endoscopy the day before POEM to assess for mucosal ulcerations or candidiasis and to clear residual food debris. Most centers do not. In the past 3 years, the authors had not had any occasion where they needed to abort a POEM procedure because of mucosal ulcerations or candidiasis and with the 5-day liquid diet, 8-hour nothing-by-mouth regimen used, there is minimal debris, that can be easily evacuated using a large-channel endoscope. The esophagus is extensively irrigated until clean. Most centers do not use antiseptic solution to clean the esophagus or gas-sterilized endoscopes. The patient is positioned supine with general anesthesia, paralysis, and positive pressure ventilation. POEM is performed in an operating room by most centers and an endoscopy room by few centers. Because of space limitations a detailed presentation of equipment and technique is not provided here. A detailed narrated video exposition of the equipment and technique along with technique variations, tips, and tricks is provided elsewhere (Video Journal and Encyclopedia of GI Endoscopy accepted for publication manuscript# VJGIEN-D-12-00541R1). An abridged presentation follows.

Equipment

Necessary equipment includes

1. Diagnostic gastroscope, preferably high resolution with accessory irrigation channel
2. Clear distal cap attachment (the authors use the 4-mm straight Olympus cap, Center Valley, PA, USA, and secure it with water resistant tape; other centers use tapered caps or oblique caps by Olympus)

Table 2
Comparing selected published POEM experiences by site: patient population and procedural data

Sites	Yokohama, Japan[32]	Rome, Italy[33]	Portland, Oregon[34]	Hamburg and Frankfurt, Germany; Amsterdam, the Netherlands; Zürich, Switzerland; Montreal, Canada[35]	Hamburg and Frankfurt, Germany[36]	Yokohama, Japan[37]	Mineola, New York[30]	Shanghai, China[38]
Number of centers	1	1	1	5	2	1	1	1
Number of patients	17	11	5	51	16	236[a]	12	205
Completed POEMs	17	10	5	51	16	236[a]	12	202
Age, mean y (range)	41.4 (18–62)	32 (24–58)	67[b] (49–78)	43 (20–76)	45 (26–76)	—(3–87)	51 (24–73)	43.9 (6–75)
Gender (female: male)	7:10	8:3	2:3	22:29	4:12	—	5:7	—
Duration of achalasia, mo (range)	100.8 (6–360)	21.5	—	—	—	132 (6–600)	52 (2–240)	104.4 (3–600)
Type of Achalasia								
Nonsigmoid (N)	12 N	10 N	5 N	—	—	16 S	9 N	—
Sigmoid (S)	5 S	0 S	0 S	—	—	—	3 S	—

Esophageal Diameter								
Grade I (<3.5 cm)	3	—	0	—	—	—	—	1
Grade II (3.5–6 cm)	11	—	—	—	—	—	—	9
Grade III (>6 cm)	3	—	—	—	—	—	—	2
Prior treatment								
Botox (BT)	—	1 BT	4 BT	—	1 BT	—	—	0 BT
Dilation (PD)	3PD	1 PD	1 PD	—	9 PD	—	—	0 PD
BTI + PD	—	—	—	—	1 BT + PD	—	—	—
Heller (HM)	—	—	—	—	—	5 HM	—	0 HM
Procedure time, mean min (range)	126 (100–180)	100.7 (75–140)	105 (57–237)	(120–240)	114 (65–188)	113.4 (56–240)	150 (102–240)	68.5 (10–180)
Length of myotomy, mean cm (range)	8.1 N: 6.5 (3–14) S: 10.6 (7–15)	10.2	7.5[b] (6–12)	13 (7–23)	12 (8–17)	14 (3–23)	5.5 (3–10)	9.5 (7–13)
Length of stay, mean d (range)	4.8 (3–8)	4	1.2	—	—	5.9 (3–10)	—	2.2 (1–4)

[a] Total number per communication with lead author (Eleftheriadis).
[b] Median.

3. Triangular tip (TT) ESD knife (Olympus; **Fig. 2**) or T-type hybrid knife (HK) (ERBE Elektromedizin GmbH, Tubingen, Germany; **Fig. 3**) (requires ERBEjet pump)
4. High-frequency electrosurgical generator (eg, ERBE VIO 300D)
5. Coagulation graspers (Olympus)
6. Endoscopic clips for closure of mucosotomy and any mucosal injuries (eg, Resolution clip, Boston Scientific, Natick, MA, USA; EZ clip or Quick-clip from Olympus).
7. Needle for decompression of capnoperitoneum if necessary (angiocath or Veress needle).
8. Optional: balloon for submucosal tunnel initiation or extension (the authors have used esophageal or pyloric dilation balloons or short-nosed biliary extraction balloons 10 to 12 mm in size, from various manufacturers).

Technique

A graphic illustration of the major POEM technique steps is shown in **Fig. 4**. Endoscopic images illustrating the steps of the POEM technique are shown in **Fig. 5**.

1. A submucosal injection is used to expand the submucosal space 10 to 15 cm proximal to the LES followed by a 2-cm long mucosal incision.
2. The endoscope is inserted into the submucosal space and with sequential submucosal injection and submucosal dissection using an electrical knife, a dilation balloon, or a combination thereof, a long submucosal tunnel is created along the right wall of the esophagus and is extended beyond the LES 2 to 3 cm into the submucosa of the cardia.
3. The endoscope is then withdrawn to approximately 2 to 3 cm distal to the mucosal incision site where the start of the myotomy takes place, thus offsetting the mucosal defect and the muscle defect (which is the ingenious feature of this technique that allows secure closure). At the start of the myotomy, the muscle is dissected until the plane between the inner circular and outer longitudinal layer is exposed. At that point, the circular muscle myotomy is initiated by hooking the circular fibers with the knife and cutting them proceeding distally until the myotomy is extended about 1 to 2 cm into the cardia (cardiomyotomy). Extension of the myotomy to the muscle of the cardia is based largely on LHM literature demonstrating higher efficacy of HM when it includes cardiomyotomy.[42] A small recent study in a porcine survival model suggested that this may also be the case with POEM.[43] Recognizing the gastroesophageal junction (GEJ) and cardia while in the tunnel can be challenging. Useful indicators of the GEJ and cardia are listed in **Box 1**. Some of the more challenging indicators to recognize by novice POEM operators are illustrated with endoscopic pictures (**Fig. 6**).

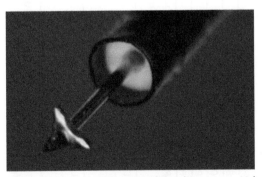

Fig. 2. Triangular tip knife (Olympus). (*Courtesy of* Haruhiro Inoue, Yokohama, Japan.)

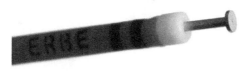

Fig. 3. T-type hybrid knife (ERBE Elektromedizin). Note the tiny injection port at the tip of the knife, which allows saline injection during dissection. (*Courtesy of* ERBE, Marietta, GA.)

It should be emphasized that POEM is a technique in evolution. For example, at the beginning of the authors' experience in 2009, no specialized ESD knives were available in the United States. Furthermore, their experience with ESD, the technique encompassing the critical skills required for POEM, although extensive by Western standards, was limited by Asian standards (a common handicap of Western

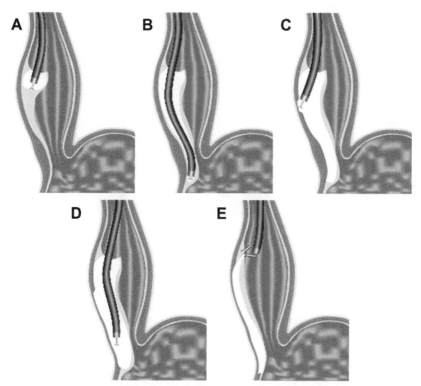

Fig. 4. POEM technique. (*A*) After submucosal (SM) saline injection, a mucosotomy is performed and dissection of the SM tunnel is initiated. (*B*) Dissection of SM tunnel is extended to the gastric cardia. (*C*) Myotomy initiation. Dissection of the circular layer. (*D*) Extension of the myotomy to the muscle of the cardia with approximately 2-cm long cardiomyotomy. (*E*) Closure of the mucosotomy (entrance to the SM tunnel) using endoscopic clips. (*Courtesy of* Winthrop University Hospital, Mineola, NY).

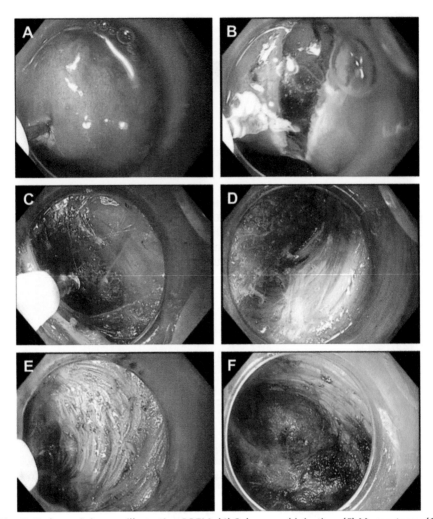

Fig. 5. Endoscopic images illustrating POEM. (*A*) Submucosal injection. (*B*) Mucosotomy. (*C*) Initiation of submucosal tunnel dissection. (*D*) Tunnel extended to gastroesophageal junction (GEJ) (note aberrant inner longitudinal fibers). (*E*) Dissection over LES. (*F*) Dissection successfully extended into cardia (note wider submucosal space and larger coagulated vessels at 5-o'clock). (*G*) LES clasp fibers as seen after completion of submucosal tunnel. (*H*) Initiation of myotomy (note circular muscle fibers). (*I*) Dissection has reached the plane between circular and longitudinal fibers, circular myotomy initiated. (*J*) Completed myotomy, the cut edges of the muscle are seen at 2 o'clock and 5 o'clock. (*K*) Submucosal tunnel entry site before closure. (*L*) Complete closure of submucosal tunnel site with endoclips.

endoscopists). For these reasons, they used a variant technique with blunt tunnel dissection using only a dilation balloon (rather than electrosurgical dissection with a dedicated ESD knife, as described by Inoue),[28] and they performed the myotomy using a traditional plain needle knife.[29] The balloon dilation approach results in faster tunnel formation but requires care during blunt insertion of the balloon catheter in the submucosa to avoid injury of the mucosa or muscularis propria. After dedicated ESD

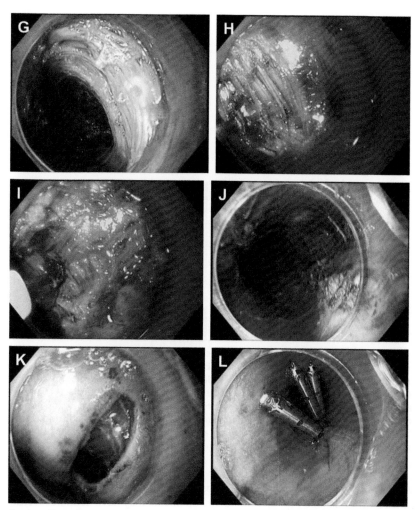

Fig. 5. (continued)

Box 1
Confirmation of tunnel extension through the GEJ into the cardia

1. Depth of insertion from incisors (centimeter marks on endoscope)
2. Resistance to endoscope insertion at the level of the sphincter
3. Wider submucosal space with large perforating vessels in the cardia
4. Blue discoloration of the cardia mucosa seen on retroflexion (from the blue dye used in the submucosal injectate)
5. Palisading vessels on the underside of the mucosal flap present at GEJ
6. Spindle-like veins in the submucosa and muscularis at the GEJ
7. Bundles of aberrant inner longitudinal muscle fibers running in the submucosa and inserting into the circular layer of the muscularis propria

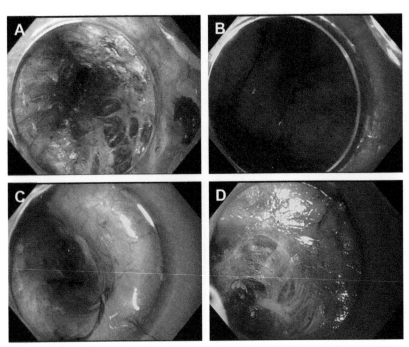

Fig. 6. Four identifiers of the GEJ/cardia. (*A*) Long, thin "palisading vessels" are seen on the underside of the mucosa at the level of the GEJ at 7-o'clock to 11-o'clock. (*B*) Blue discoloration of the cardia mucosa is seen on retroflexion (from the blue dye used in the submucosal injectate) after the submucosal tunnel is successfully extended to the cardia. (*C*) Spindle-like veins in the submucosa and muscularis are present at the level of the GEJ. (*D*) Bundles of aberrant inner longitudinal muscle fibers running in the submucosa and inserting into the circular layer of the muscularis propria is another marker that the level of the GEJ has been reached.

knives became available in the United States, the authors started using the TT knife as described by Inoue (see **Fig. 2**). For the last 25 cases, they have used the T-type HK (see **Fig. 3**) for submucosal dissection and myotomy without any recourse to balloon dilation. Based on their experience involving use of the TT knife in 11 cases and the HK in 25 cases, the ability of the HK to perform submucosal injection without need for continual exchange between needle injector and knife (as is the case with the TT knife) may increase dissection safety and speed. Zhou and coworkers[44] compared the HK and TT knife in a head-to-head prospective randomized study. The results, reported in abstract form, revealed shorter procedure time, lower bleeding rate, and less frequent usage of coagulation forceps with the HK. The mean duration of POEM (see **Table 2**) is approximately 90 to 120 minutes. Incredibly, procedure times as short as 10 minutes were reported by the Shanghai group where the main operator, Professor Zhou, has performed over 300 POEMs. POEM duration is very sensitive to case difficulty and thus prone to wide fluctuation as can be inferred, for example, from the range of procedure times between 10 and 180 minutes in the data from Shanghai. In the authors' series, most POEMs were completed in 2 hours or less but several POEMs extended to as long as 4 hours in challenging cases with extremely high LES pressures, severe sigmoidization, megaesophagus, and prior BTI or LHM.

COMPLICATIONS AND MANAGEMENT

Data regarding adverse events (AE) remain limited. The authors have had no signifi-cant AEs in the 43 POEMs they have performed to date despite having included patients as old as 93, patients with significant comorbidities including emphysema and heart failure, patients with end-stage achalasia, patients with prior PD-BTI, and a patient with failed LHM. Minor AEs included tense capnoperitoneum and inadvertent injuries to the mucosal flap in a small number of patients early in their experience easily treated with needle decompression and placement of endoscopic clips, respectively, without any significant clinical impact. AEs are listed in **Table 3** for published series and in **Table 4** for IPOEMS. In the publication by Ren and colleagues[40] the very high rate of pneumothorax of about 28% is at variance with all other series and, along with the very high rates of pneumoperitoneum and subcutaneous and mediastinal emphysema, is believed to be caused by this group's initial use of air instead of CO_2 for insufflation. Use of CO_2 is essential to minimize such complications. Severe nonfatal AEs were reported in about 3% of patients in IPOEMS (see **Table 4**) consist-ing mostly of bleeding in the tunnel or pneumothorax and related chest morbidity. There was a single reported patient with a paraesophageal abscess in the IPOEMS data but no reported instances of leaks and mediastinal sepsis, the initial paramount concern of most investigators embarking on POEM. No mortality has been reported but there is a rumored death of a 19-year-old woman from mediastinal sepsis after POEM. This rather alarming rumor has not been confirmed at this time several months since its first appearance.[45] It should be noted that if this event is confirmed, and assuming that there are no other unreported deaths at this time, this would put POEM mortality at approximately 1 per 900, similar to the 0.0% to 0.8% mortality of LHM.[46]

POSTOPERATIVE CARE

Most centers perform a contrast esophagram to exclude a leak and discharge the patient 1 to 2 days after POEM. Few centers outside the United States keep patients in the hospital as long as 5 to 7 days. Half of the 16 IPOEMS participating centers perform a "second look" endoscopy before discharge but this endoscopy yields actionable findings very infrequently and may not be a cost-effective intervention. Despite not performing "second look endoscopy" and discharging patients at a median of 2 days, the authors have not had any postdischarge POEM complications or readmissions to date. Much less pain than in LHM has been noted in the authors' series with only 14% requiring any narcotics postoperatively. This has also been the experience of other POEM operators.[34,36]

OUTCOMES

Table 5 presents data from published series on the impressive overall POEM treatment success rate and significant improvements in mean LES pressure and mean symptom score (most series use the Eckardt score, **Table 6**). Even with the caveats of small numbers, early experience, and short-term follow-up, the universally reported POEM treatment success of greater than 90% is similar to the initial treatment success of LHM.[46] In the authors' series of 43 patients, all attempted POEMs were successfully and safely completed despite the significant number of high-risk complex patients. For the 29 patients for whom minimum follow-up of at least 3 months is available, the mean Eckardt score improved from 7.41 before POEM to 1 after POEM (*P*<.0001). There have been only 2 out of 29 failures (Eckardt score >3) for an overall success

Table 3
Adverse events reported in published POEM series

	Adverse Events		
Study	Intraoperative No. of Cases (%)	Postoperative No. of Cases (%)	Follow-Up No. of Cases (%)
Costamagna (10 cases)	Junctional flap perforation 2/10 (20%) Cervical emphysema 2/10 (20%) Pneumomediastinum 10/10 (100%)	Mild chest pain 10/10 (100%)	—
von Renteln (16 cases)	Full-thickness dissection into peritoneal cavity 9/16 (56.3%) Full-thickness dissection into mediastinum 13/16 (81.3%)	Cutaneous emphysema 6/16 (37.5%) Pneumoperitoneum 8/16 (50%) Mucosal perforation 1/16 (6.3%) Superficial ulcer at cardia 1/16 (6.3%) Ulcer in distal esophagus 1/16 (6.3%)	Erosive esophagitis 1/16 (6.3%)
Yoshida (161 cases)	—	Aspiration pneumonia 1/161 (0.6%) Lesser omentum inflammation 1/161 (0.6%) Submucosal hematoma 1/161 (0.6%) Pneumothorax 1/161 (0.6%)	GERD 17/161 (10.6%)
Eleftheriadis (236 cases)	—	Local peritonitis 1/197 (0.5%) Mucosal laceration in cardia 3/197 (1.5%) Intramucosal hematoma 1/197 (0.5%) Pneumothorax 1/197 (0.5%)	—
Ren (119 cases)	Cutaneous emphysema 27/119 (22.7%) Pneumothorax 3/119 (2.5%)	Pneumothorax 30/119 (25.2%) Subcutaneous emphysema 66/119 (55.5%) Mediastinal emphysema 35/119 (29.4%) Delayed hemorrhage 1/119 (0.8%) Pleural effusion 58/119 (48.7%) Segmental atelectasis of the lungs 59/119 (49.6%) Aeroperitoneum 47/119 (39.5%)	Esophageal stricture 1/119 (0.8%) Dehiscence at tunnel entry 1/119 (0.8%)
Swanstrom (5 cases)	Gastric mucosotomies 2/5 (40%) Pneumoperitoneum 3/5 (60%)	—	—

Table 4	
IPOEMS reported adverse events	
International POEM Survey (IPOEMS) Data: Adverse Events	
Total number/percent of patients with any severe nonfatal AEs[a]	27 (3.2%)
Interventional radiology/nonsurgical invasive procedures to correct AEs	16 (1.9%)
Intensive care unit admissions	10 (1.2%)
Hospital readmissions	9 (1.1%)
Bleeding requiring blood transfusion	8 (1%)
Cardiac arrhythmia	6 (0.7%)
Pneumonia or respiratory issue	2 (0.2%)
Mortality	0%
Minor technical AEs with minimal clinical impact	
Capnoperitoneum requiring intraprocedural venting	70 (8.3%)
Inadvertent mucosal perforation of mucosal flap	56 (6.7%)
Premature perforation of muscle layer at time of submucosal tunnel creation	20 (2.4%)

[a] Defined as follows: number of patients with AEs resulting in intensive care unit stay, readmission within 30 days, surgical conversion, surgical/IR/other intervention, prolongation of hospitalization to >5 days, intravenous antibiotics for >5 days, blood transfusions or disability requiring a higher level of care after discharge than before POEM.

rate of 93%. Both patients with treatment failure were early in the authors' experience, when they were performing shorter myotomies as initially described by Inoue and coworkers (3–5 cm).[32] Salvage PD was performed and both patients had an excellent sustained response and are currently completely asymptomatic (Eckardt score 0).

CURRENT CONTROVERSIES
Myotomy Length

The reported mean myotomy length (see **Table 2**) is 8 to 10 cm. Initial myotomies by Inoue and coworkers[32] were approximately 3 to 5 cm in length. After the safety of the technique was established, he extended them to an average of 8 to 10 cm, the recommended length in the LHM literature, and so did all other centers including the authors'. In the authors' opinion, it is now becoming increasingly apparent that myotomy length may need to be tailored to the manometric profile of the patient and that gratuitously long myotomies may offer no additional benefit in nonspastic achalasia, and may unnecessarily prolong the procedure, increase procedural risks, and even possibly subject patients to the risk of developing diveriticula through the disrupted muscle in the esophageal body.

LES Myotomy Orientation

The human LES has a complex structure[47] consisting of a weaker, thinner clasp (circular) fiber component on the lesser curvature centered at 2-o'clock (with 12-o'clock defined as the anterior-most wall on endoscopic intraluminal view) and a sling (oblique) fiber component centered on the left posterolateral wall at 7-o'clock and draping over the anterior and posterior walls to about 11- and 5-o'clock, respectively (**Fig. 7**). The sling fibers maintain the angle of His and present a significant antireflux barrier. Thus, the favorably low gastroesophageal reflux disease (GERD) rate with POEM compared with LHM may not just be caused by the fact that periesophageal ligaments with potential antireflux function, such as the phrenoesophageal membrane, are not dissected. An additional factor may be that the current 2-o'clock

Table 5
Published POEM series: outcomes

Sites	Yokohama, Japan[32]	Rome, Italy[33]	Portland, Oregon[34]	Hamburg and Frankfurt, Germany; Amsterdam, the Netherlands; Zürich, Switzerland; Montreal, Canada[35]	Hamburg and Frankfurt, Germany[36]	Yokohama, Japan[37]	Mineola, New York[30]
Number of patients	17	11	5	51 (multicenter trial)	16 (multicenter trial)	236	12
Follow-up (mo)	5	3	0.5	3	3	11[a]	9.5[a]
POEM success[b] (% of patients)	100%	91%	100%	94%	94%	99%	92%
Reason for POEM failure	—	1 case submucosal fibrosis; performed EBD	—	3 failed to have symptom improvement (Eckardt score ≤3)	1 retreatment with EBD	1 retreatment with EBD 1 retreatment with POEM	1 retreatment with EBD
Pre/post mean LES resting pressure (mm Hg), P	52.4/19.8 (P = .0001)	45.1/16.9 (P = .0)	55.1[d]/36.5[d]	27.4/10.2 (P<.001)	27.2/11.8 (P<.001)	26.8/12.6 (P<.001)	48.2/22.08 (P = .0264)
Pre/post mean Eckardt score, P	10/1.3[c] (P = .0003)	7.1/1.1 (P = .0001)	—/0 or 1[d]	7.9/1.4 (P<.001)	8.8/1.4 (P<.001)	6.36/1.45 (P = .003)	7.8/0.7 (P = .0001)
GERD symptoms	6%	0%	—	20% (7/35)	0%	10.5%	0%
GERD- endoscopic evidence (erosions)	1 reflux esophagitis LA classification B	0	—	5/30 Esophagitis	1 erosive esophagitis LA classification A	—	—

[a] Mean.

[b] Failure defined as need to use alternative achalasia treatments and failure to meet the criterion or criteria for successful treatment. It includes technical failure or inability to complete the procedure; failure to achieve appropriate symptom improvement (eg, Eckardt score ≤3); or recurrence of symptoms during the follow-up provided by these studies.

[c] Non-Eckardt dysphagia score.

[d] Median.

Table 6 Eckardt score				
		Symptoms		
Score	Weight Loss (kg)	Dysphagia	Chest Pain	Regurgitation
0	None	None	None	None
1	<5	Occasional	Occasional	Occasional
2	5–10	Daily	Daily	Daily
3	>10	Each meal	Each meal	Each meal

orientation of the POEM myotomy used by most centers results in section of the clasp fibers only and preservation of the sling fibers with their antireflux function (unlike the 11-o'clock orientation of the LHM, which results in partial transection of anterior sling fibers). One could predict that the few centers using preferentially a 5-o'clock orientation (Shanghai and the authors' team at Winthrop) or 11-o'clock (Swanstrom), thus cutting a portion of the posterior or anterior sling fibers, respectively, may have higher efficacy in dysphagia relief but possibly at the cost of increased reflux. One could envision in the future tailoring this aspect of the myotomy to disease characteristics (eg, performing a 2-o'clock "clasp fiber" myotomy in patients with low baseline LES pressures and a 5-o'clock "clasp plus partial sling" myotomy in patients with long tight LES segments or patients with unsatisfactory intraprocedural LES distensibility

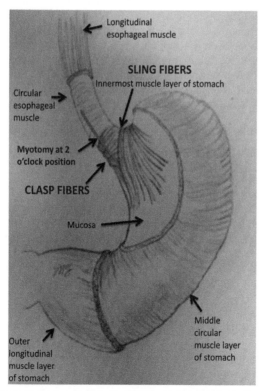

Fig. 7. Human LES anatomy in relation to POEM myotomy orientation. (*Courtesy of* S.N. Stavropoulos, Winthrop University Hospital, 2012).

assessment after a "clasp only" POEM. The authors perform such immediate assessment "qualitatively" by assessing resistance to passage of the endoscope through the LES immediately after completion of the POEM or quantitatively by obtaining intraprocedural immediate pre- and post-POEM LES distensibility measurements using the Endoflip system.[48] In one patient with poor distensibility after an initial 2-o'clock myotomy, the authors performed a second full-thickness myotomy at 5-o'clock. The functional result was excellent with an Eckardt score of 0 and widely patulous GEJ but evidence of erosive esophagitis on follow-up endoscopy associated with GERD symptoms, fortunately fully controlled on twice-daily proton pump inhibitors.

Circular Layer Myotomy Only Versus Complete Myotomy

Bonin and coworkers[43] published a randomized study in a survival pig model attempting to answer the question of whether partial or complete myotomy is more effective in lowering LES pressure. No significant decreases in postmyotomy LES pressure were seen in any group, raising concerns about technique problems. Most POEM expert centers perform partial myotomy of the circular layer and leave the longitudinal layer intact to the degree that this is possible given its relatively insubstantial nature in many patients and its propensity to "split" even with simple pressure with the endoscope. von Renteln and colleagues[36] switched from partial to complete myotomy at the cardia for the last seven patients in their published series of 16 patients. They reported rapid esophageal emptying in 83% of patients with complete myotomy versus 56% with emptying delay in the partial myotomy patients. The Shanghai group and the authors' center in New York are the only other high-volume centers favoring complete myotomy at present. The authors' preference for a complete myotomy and a more definitive 5-o'clock "clasp plus partial sling" myotomy is motivated by the belief that, at this stage, one should err on the side of efficacy rather than reflux prevention. Poor efficacy is much more detrimental to POEM development than a high rate of reflux. Proton pump inhibitors offer a very effective, simple treatment of the latter, whereas management of failed POEM with recurrent dysphagia is more problematic and is likely to have a more profound effect on patient and physician satisfaction with POEM.

Incidence of GERD after POEM

Objective endoscopic evidence of reflux has been recently reported in at least 20% of POEM patients of a European multicenter trial (see **Table 5**).[35] These concerning results are in agreement with preliminary unpublished results by the authors' group and others and are at variance with initial favorable reports[32,35,36] that depended largely on symptom assessment. This is not surprising because symptoms, as is known from the LHM literature, correlate poorly with presence of significant acid reflux in patients with achalasia. This rate of reflux is still no higher than that of LHM with fundoplication. Also, the centers in this European multicenter trial perform complete myotomy and the question again is whether by doing a complete myotomy one is trading increased efficacy for higher incidence of GERD. It is hoped that further multicenter trials will examine the impact of complete or partial myotomy and myotomy orientation on dysphagia relief and GERD. Standardization of these POEM aspects would be important before proceeding to RCTs of POEM versus other standard treatments.

FUTURE CONSIDERATIONS
Training and Accreditation

As the field moves toward POEM standardization, it should be emphasized that very large majorities of the 16 centers participating in IPOEMS supported the need for preclinical laboratory training (87.5%), proctoring on the first human cases (100%), and institutional review board approval before initiating POEM at a center (62.5%). There was also very high agreement in recommending formal center accreditation for POEM ("similar to that used for bariatric surgery centers in the US") (68.8%); POEM operator certification ("similar to that used for robotic surgery in the US") (68.8%); and mandatory reporting of severe AE to an independent monitoring body (87.5%). The strong agreement with regard to these recommendations despite the disparate backgrounds of respondents (including surgeons and gastroenterologists across Asia, Europe, and North America) underscores the fact that POEM is an invasive endoscopic surgical procedure that requires appropriate training and preparation, and rigorous accreditation and monitoring of outcomes to ensure safety and efficacy.

Table 7
Retrospective comparison of POEM to LHM

	POEM	LHM	P
Number of patients	11	50	
Age (y)	36 ± 11 (18–85)	50 ± 16	$P<.01$
Prior achalasia treatment	None	—	
Type of achalasia	11 nonsigmoid	—	
Gender (male: female)	7: 4	26: 24	ns
Duration of symptoms (y)	2 ± 5	2 ± 3	ns
Operation time (min)	121 ± 42	126 ± 29	ns
Estimated blood loss (mL)	≤10	91 ± 55	$P<.001$
Myotomy length (cm)	8 ± 1.1	8.5 ± 0.7	$P = .04$
Pain score on day of surgery	3.3 ± 3.1	2.1 ± 2.3	ns
Pain score on postoperative Day 1	2.5 ± 2.8	2.1 ± 2.3	ns
Use of narcotics on day of surgery (mg morphine equivalents)	4.8 ± 5.2	2.8 ± 4.3	ns
Use of narcotics on postoperative Day 1 (mg morphine equivalents)	6.9 ± 7.7	4.6 ± 5	ns
Length of hospitalization (d)	2.3 ± 3.6	1.6 ± 2.9	ns
Minor complication, number of cases	3 (27%)	7 (14%)	ns
Major complication	A contained leak at the EGJ requiring laparoscopic drain placement	Delayed esophageal leak requiring thoracotomy for drainage and repair	
Preoperative vs 6-wk postoperative LES basal and relaxation pressure (mm Hg)	Basal: 25 ± 10 vs 12 ± 7 — Relaxation: 29 ± 17 vs 15 ± 3	—	$P = .04$ $P<.05$
Timed barium: difference in contrast height (cm) at 1, 2, and 5 min	4 vs 17 2 vs 16 2 vs 11	—	$P = .02$ $P = .04$

Data from Hungness E, Teitelbaum E, Santos B, et al. Comparison of perioperative outcomes after per-oral esophageal myotomy (POEM) and laparoscopic Heller myotomy. Gastroenterology 2012;142(Suppl 1):S1035–6.

Niche of POEM in Achalasia Therapy and Implications Regarding Future RCTs

Two POEM centers where POEM is performed by surgeons with significant prior experience with LHM, one in Germany and one in the United States, have presented in lectures archived online unpublished data comparing recent consecutive LHMs to the initial experience with POEM by the same operators that performed the LHMs.[49,50] Both series revealed similar results. In the interest of time and space only the results by Hungness and colleagues[50] are presented (**Table 7**). Although these are relatively low-quality retrospective data, they seem to suggest at least equivalence in operative time, morbidity, and efficacy. This center's narcotic requirement, for unclear reasons, is higher than that of most other centers as reviewed previously. These are very encouraging data because equivalence at this point, with POEM being at a nascent stage and LHM at a mature, fully developed stage, likely portends dominance of the less invasive POEM in the not too distant future. Based on the data reviewed here, it is not surprising that most POEM experts, including surgeons with extensive LHM experience, believe that POEM will achieve results as durable as those of LHM but with less invasiveness similar to that of endoscopic therapies and thus largely replace LHM. POEM could plausibly become the first-line treatment approach for achalasia in all patients except those with very severe comorbidities or end-stage sigmoid esophagus or megaesophagus.

In view of these auspicious forecasts and fairly enthusiastic adoption of POEM within the achalasia patient community, it seems that it would probably not be feasible or ultimately even clinically relevant to attempt to enroll patients in an RCT comparing POEM to LHM. It seems that the most relevant and feasible study would be a head-to-head comparison of POEM and PD with cross-over of failures.

Offshoots of POEM

POEM is spawning a brave new world of endoluminal surgery using the technique of submucosal tunneling. New procedures being developed range from pyloromyotomy[51] to full-thickness en bloc resection of subepithelial tumors of the esophagus and GEJ, locations poorly accessible to surgery.[52,53]

SUMMARY

POEM clearly is a paradigm shift in achalasia therapy where essentially an endoscopic procedure with its associated convenience and less invasiveness can duplicate clinical results of a time-tested surgical procedure (LHM). Further refinements of the POEM technique are expected.

REFERENCES

1. Spechler SJ, Souza RF, Rosenberg SJ, et al. Heartburn in patients with achalasia. Gut 2005;37:305–8.
2. Mayberry JF. Epidemiology and demographics of achalasia. Gastrointest Endosc Clin N Am 2001;11:235–48.
3. Richter JE. Achalasia-an update. J Neurogastroenterol Motil 2010;16(3):232–42.
4. Duranceau A, Liberman M, Martin J, et al. End-stage achalasia. Dis Esophagus 2012;25(4):319–30.
5. Walzer N, Hirano I. Achalasia. Gastroenterol Clin North Am 2008;37(4):807–25, viii.
6. Zerbid F, Thetiot V, Richy F, et al. Repeated pneumatic dilations as long-term maintenance therapy for esophageal achalasia. Am J Gastroenterol 2006; 101(4):692–7.

7. Parkman HP, Reynolds JC, Ouyang A, et al. Pneumatic dilation or esophagomyotomy for idiopathic achalasia: clinical outcomes and cost analysis. Dig Dis Sci 1993;38(1):75–85.
8. Bravi I, Nicita MT, Duca P, et al. A pneumatic dilation strategy in achalasia: prospective outcome and effects on oesophageal motor function in the long term. Aliment Pharmacol Ther 2010;31(6):658–65.
9. Kadakia SC, Wong RH. Graded pneumatic dilation using Rigiflex achalasia dilators in patients with primary esophageal achalasia. Am J Gastroenterol 1993;88: 34–8.
10. Borotto E, Gaudric M, Daniel B, et al. Risk factors for immediate complications after progressive pneumatic dilation for achalasia. Gut 1996;39(1):9–12.
11. Pretap N, Kalapala R, Darrissetty S, et al. Achalasia cardia subtyping by high-resolution manometry predicts the therapeutic outcome of pneumatic balloon dilatation. J Neurogastroenterol Motil 2011;17(1):48–53.
12. Boeckxstaens GE, Annese V, des Varannes SB, et al. Pneumatic dilation versus laparoscopic Heller's myotomy for idiopathic achalasia. N Engl J Med 2011; 364(19):1807–16.
13. Pasricha PJ, Ravich WJ, Hendrix TR, et al. Intrasphincteric botulinum for the treatment of achalasia. N Engl J Med 1995;332(12):774–8.
14. Pasricha PJ, Rai R, Ravich WJ, et al. Botulinum toxin for achalasia: long term outcome and predictors of response. Gastroenterology 1996;110(5):1410–5.
15. Annese V, Bassotti G, Coccia G, et al. A multicentre randomized study of intrasphincteric botulinum toxin in patients with oesophageal achalasia. GISMAD achalasia study group. Gut 2000;46(5):587–600.
16. Lake JM, Wong RH. Review article: the management of achalasia-a comparison of different treatment modalities. Aliment Pharmacol Ther 2006;24(6):909–20.
17. Enestvedt BK, Williams JL, Sonnenberg A. Epidemiology and practice patterns of achalasia in a large multi-centre database. Aliment Pharmacol Ther 2011;33(11): 1209–14.
18. Niknam R, Mikael J, Mehrabi N, et al. Ethanolamine oleate in resistant idiopathic achalasia: a novel therapy. Eur J Gastroenterol Hepatol 2011;23(12):1111–5.
19. De Palma GD, Iovino P, Masone S, et al. Self-expanding metal stents for endoscopic treatment of achalasia unresponsive to conventional treatments. Long term results in eight patients. Endoscopy 2001;33(12):1027–30.
20. Mukherjee S, Kaplan DS, Parasher G, et al. Expandable metal stents in achalasia-is there a role? Am J Gastroenterol 2000;95(9):2185–8.
21. Li YD, Tang GY, Cheng YS, et al. 13-year follow-up of a prospective comparison of the long-term clinical efficacy of temporary self-expanding metallic stents and pneumatic dilation for the treatment of achalasia in 120 patients. AJR Am J Roentgenol 2010;195(6):1429–37.
22. Zhao JG, Li YD, Cheng YS, et al. Long term safety and outcome of a temporary self-expanding metal stent for achalasia: a prospsective study with a 13 year experience. Eur Radiol 2009;19(8):1973–80.
23. Li YD, Cheng YS, Li MH, et al. Temporary self-expanding metal stents and pneumatic dilation for the treatment of achalasia: a prospective study with long-term follow-up. Dis Esophagus 2010;23(5):361–7.
24. Cheng YS, Ma F, Li YD, et al. Temporary self-expanding metallic stents for achalasia: a prospective study with long term follow-up. World J Gastroenterol 2010; 16(40):5111–7.
25. Dua KS. Expandable stents for benign esophageal disease. Gastrointest Endosc 2011;21(3):359–76.

26. Sumiyama K, Gostout CJ, Rajan E, et al. Transesophageal mediastinoscopy by submucosal endoscopy with mucosal flap safety valve technique. Gastrointest Endosc 2007;65(4):679–83.

27. Pasricha PJ, Hawari R, Ahmed I, et al. Submucosal endoscopic esophageal myotomy: a novel experimental approach for the treatment of achalasia. Endoscopy 2007;39(9):761–4.

28. Inoue H, Minami H, Satodate H, et al. First clinical experience of submucosal endoscopic myotomy for esophageal achalasia with no skin incision (with video). Gastrointest Endosc 2009;69(5):AB122.

29. Stavropoulos SN, Harris MD, Hida S, et al. Endoscopic submucosal myotomy for the treatment of achalasia (with video). Gastrointest Endosc 2010;72(6): 1309–11.

30. Stavropoulos SN, Brathwaite C, Iqbal S, et al. POEM (peroral endoscopic myotomy), a US gastroenterologist perspective: initial 2 year experience. Gastrointest Endosc 2012;75(4):AB149.

31. Shiwaku H, Inoue H, Beppu R, et al. Successful treatment of diffuse esophageal spasm by per oral endoscopic myotomy. Gastrointest Endosc 2012. http://dx.doi.org/10.1016/j.gie.2012.02.008.

32. Inoue H, Minami H, Kobayashi Y, et al. Per oral endoscopic myotomy (POEM) for esophageal achalasia. Endoscopy 2010;42(4):265–71.

33. Costamagna G, Marchese M, Familiari P, et al. Peroral endoscopic myotomy (POEM) for oesophageal achalasia: preliminary results in humans. Dig Liver Dis 2012;44(10):827–32.

34. Swanstrom LL, Rieder E, Dunst CM. A stepwise approach and early clinical experience in Per oral endoscopic myotomy for the treatment of achalasia and esophageal motility disorders. J Am Coll Surg 2011;213(6):751–6.

35. von Renteln D, Fuchs KH, Fockens P, et al. Per oral endoscopic myotomy for the treatment of achalasia: prospective international multi center study. Gastrointest Endosc 2012;75(4S):AB160.

36. von Renteln D, Inoue H, Minami H, et al. Per oral endoscopic myotomy for the treatment of achalasia: a prospective single center study. Am J Gastroenterol 2012;107(3):411–7.

37. Eleftheriadis N, Inoue H, Ikeda H, et al. Training in peroral endoscopic myotomy (POEM) for esophageal achalasia. Ther Clin Risk Manag 2012;8:329–42.

38. Zhou P, Yao L, Zhang YQ, et al. Per oral endoscopic myotomy (POEM) for esophageal achalasia: 205 cases report. Gastrointest Endosc 2012;75(4): AB132–3.

39. Inoue H, Tianle KM, Ikeda H, et al. Peroral endoscopic myotomy for esophageal achalasia: technique, indication, and outcomes. Thorac Surg Clin 2011;21(4): 519–25.

40. Ren Z, Zhong Y, Zhou P, et al. Perioperative management and treatment for complications during and after peroral endoscopic myotomy (POEM) for esophageal achalasia (EA) (data from 119 cases). Surg Endosc 2012;26(11): 3267–72.

41. Stefanidis D, Richardson W, Farrell T, et al. SAGES guidelines for the surgical treatment of esophageal achalasia. Surg Endosc 2012;26(2):296–311.

42. Oelschlager BK, Chang L, Pellegrini CA. Improved outcome after extended gastric myotomy for achalasia. Arch Surg 2003;138:490–5.

43. Bonin EA, Moran E, Bingener J, et al. A comparative study of endoscopic full-thickness and partial-thickness myotomy using submucosal endoscopy with mucosal safety flap (SEMF) technique. Surg Endosc 2012;26:1751–8.

44. Zhou P, Yao L, Cai M, et al. Water-jet assisted per oral endoscopic myotomy (POEM) in comparison to conventional endoscopic myotomy technique for treatment of esophageal achalasia. Gastrointest Endosc 2012;75(4):AB160–1.
45. Swanstrom L. POEM: North American experience. Presented at the SAGES 2012 Conference PG course per oral endoscopic myotomy (POEM). San Diego, March 8, 2012.
46. Campos GM, Vittinghoff E, Rabl C, et al. Endoscopic and surgical treatments for achalasia: a systematic review and meta-analysis. Ann Surg 2009;249(1):45–57.
47. Stein HJ, Liebermann-Meffert D, DeMeester TR, et al. Three dimensional pressure image and muscular structure of the human lower esophageal sphincter. Surgery 1995;17:692–8.
48. Rohof WO, Hirsch DP, Kessing BF, et al. Efficacy of treatment for patients with achalasia depends on the distensibility of the esophagogastric junction. Gastroenterology 2012;143(2):328–35.
49. Fuchs KH. Postgraduate course: per oral endoscopic myotomy (POEM): clinical experience in Europe. Presented at SAGES 2012 Meeting, San Diego, March 8, 2012.
50. Hungness E, Teitelbaum E, Santos B, et al. Comparison of perioperative outcomes after per-oral esophageal myotomy (POEM) and laparoscopic Heller myotomy. Gastroenterology 2012;142(5):S1035–6 Supplement 1.
51. Kawai M, Peretta S, Burckhardt O, et al. Endoscopic pyloromyotomy: a new concept of minimally invasive surgery for pyloric stenosis. Endoscopy 2012;44: 169–73.
52. Xu MD, Cai MY, Zhou PH, et al. Submucosal tunneling endoscopic resection: a new technique for treating upper GI submucosal tumors originating from the muscularis propria layer. Gastrointest Endosc 2012;75:195–9.
53. Inoue H, Ikeda H, Hosoya T, et al. Submucosal endoscopic tumor resection for subepithelial tumors in the esophagus and cardia. Endoscopy 2012;44:225–30.

Early Gastric Cancer and Dysplasia

Wataru Tamura, MD, Norio Fukami, MD*

KEYWORDS

- Early gastric cancer • Endoscopic mucosal resection
- Endoscopic submucosal dissection • Lymph node dissection
- Laparoscopic gastrectomy

KEY POINTS

- Gastric adenomas are a precursor for early gastric cancer (EGC) and patients should undergo endoscopic resection followed by appropriate surveillance.
- Endoscopic resection of EGC has become the preferred therapeutic procedure within the appropriate criteria, and it provides the most accurate tumor staging and risk assessment for lymph node metastasis.
- Endoscopic submucosal dissection allows resection in a wider range of patients, and the criteria have expanded for endoscopic treatment.
- A less invasive surgical approach has been investigated, yielding promising results for nonendoscopic resection candidates and noncurative endoscopic resections.

INTRODUCTION

Gastric adenocarcinoma is the second leading cause of global cancer mortality, with nearly 1 million cases annually. Gastric cancer has marked geographic and ethnic variability (with high-incidence areas in Eastern Asia, Latin America, parts of Europe, and the Middle East,[1] and increased rates in certain ethnic groups such as Asians, Hispanics, and African Americans).[2] In Western countries, early gastric cancer (EGC) accounts only for 15% to 21% of gastric cancer.[3] Early detection is particularly important, because EGC has a much better prognosis than more advanced stages of gastric adenocarcinoma, with a 5-year survival rate of approximately 90%. EGC is defined as gastric cancer that invades the mucosa and submucosa, irrespective of lymph node metastases (T1, any N),[4] and is of particular importance in Eastern Asia. In Japan, the incidence of EGC is higher than in the western population anywhere, from 15% to as high as 57%,[5–7] because screening programs were implemented many decades ago.

Division of Gastroenterology & Hepatology, University of Colorado Denver Anschutz Medical Campus, 12631 East 17th Avenue, Mailstop B-158, Academic Office 1, Aurora, CO 80045, USA
* Corresponding author.
E-mail address: norio.fukami@ucdenver.edu

Gastrointest Endoscopy Clin N Am 23 (2013) 77–94
http://dx.doi.org/10.1016/j.giec.2012.10.011
1052-5157/13/$ – see front matter © 2013 Elsevier Inc. All rights reserved.

giendo.theclinics.com

Consideration for the Treatment of EGC

EGC was first described in Japan in 1962, and it was defined as a neoplasm that could be successfully treated with surgery. Later, it was internationally defined more specifically as gastric adenocarcinoma that is restricted to the mucosa and submucosa irrespective of lymph node metastases (T1, any N).[4] The ongoing debate regarding whether nodal metastatic disease should still be considered "early" gastric cancer stems from the difficulty in selecting appropriate candidates for endoscopic resection versus gastrectomy, which removes regional lymph nodes.[3] Some patients with EGC are at high risk for nodal metastases and are not appropriate for endoscopic resection. However, preremoval image-based assessment to determine the need for surgical therapy was proven to be less accurate than postendoscopic removal histologic assessment. Thus, endoscopic resection with intent to cure is often considered the final staging assessment to stratify patients who would benefit from more invasive surgical therapy. In summary, as worldwide experience in endoscopic resection continues to grow and provide further evidence (including comparative studies with surgical treatments), the criteria for endoscopic therapy is expected to expand.

PRETREATMENT EVALUATION

Macroscopic description of early gastrointestinal neoplasia (EGN), including dysplasia and cancer, was summarized in the Vienna classification of gastrointestinal epithelial neoplasia[8] and the Japanese macroscopic classification of superficial gastric carcinoma (Japan Gastroenterological Endoscopy Society [JGES] classification system),[9] from which an international consensus system was proposed in 2002 called the *Paris system*,[10] underscoring the importance of these classifications. Gastric adenoma, defined as intraepithelial or noninvasive gastric dysplasia, progresses in an unpredictable time frame from low-grade to high-grade dysplasia or carcinoma in situ, and to invasive neoplasia (adenocarcinoma). High-grade dysplasia is a direct precursor to invasive cancer, with a known risk for associated synchronous cancer, and therefore a treatment is indicated and the remainder of the stomach must be carefully examined.[11–14] Endoscopic resection is recommended for all gastric adenomas because of the risk for transformation to adenocarcinoma.

Endoscopic detection of EGN requires meticulous evaluation and photodocumentation of lesions.[15] Their appearance varies widely, and can include a subtle polypoid protrusion, a superficial plaque, ulcer, depression, or even a mucosal discoloration.[16] Novel endoscopic imaging technologies have been investigated to improve detection, including chromoendoscopy,[17,18] magnification endoscopy, special image acquisition or processing (eg, narrow band imaging [NBI]), and autofluorescence imaging.[19–24] Endoscopic findings can predict tumor stage and depth of invasion of EGN. Mucosal disease is suggested by smooth surface protrusion or depression, slight marginal elevation, and smooth tapering of converging folds, whereas submucosal disease is indicated by an irregular surface, marked marginal elevation, clubbing, abrupt cutting, or fusion of converging folds.[25] Tumor factors associated with lymph node metastasis derived from "*histological*" data are summarized in **Box 1**.[26–30]

ENDOSCOPIC ULTRASOUND

Endoscopic ultrasound (EUS) is the most reliable nonhistopathologic method for evaluating the invasion depth of gastric cancer, allowing visualization of the gastric wall

---

Box 1
Factors associated with lymph node metastasis

- Large tumor size (>20, especially >30 mm)
- Diffuse (undifferentiated) or mixed (intestinal/undifferentiated) histology
- Ulceration
- Submucosal involvement (especially >0.5 mm)
- Lymphovascular invasion

---

layers.[31] T-stage determination with EUS is more accurate than computed tomography (CT) scanning for gastric cancer,[32,33] and EUS-guided fine-needle aspiration of suspicious nodes has increased the accuracy of nodal staging. The limitations of EUS are that the staging accuracy is limited in separating among T1m and T1sm 1 through 3, and it varies with the size, location, and differentiation of the tumor (eg, overstaged with inflammation when >3 cm and located in the mid-stomach, and understaged with poorly differentiated tumors).[34] EUS is used less for pretreatment evaluation of EGC, because endoscopic findings and the postendoscopic resection specimen can guide treatment.[35]

TREATMENT OPTIONS
Endoscopic Resection

Endoscopic mucosal resection
Polypectomy was first introduced in 1968, and endoscopic mucosal resection (EMR) has emerged and evolved since the 1980s. It is an alternative to gastrectomy for patients who meet the standard criteria for endoscopic resection of EGC.[36] Historical standard criteria for EMR according to JGES was protruded lesions equal or less than 2 cm, flat or depressed lesions equal or less than 1cm and the cancers limited to mucosa (**Box 2**).[37,38] A review of the Japanese literature showed that an extremely high rate of disease-specific survival is achieved when the JGES criteria for EMR are satisfied (>99% among 1353 patients followed up for 4 months to 11 years).[39] In addition, both Japanese and Western studies have shown high survival rates in patients with EGC treated with EMR, with a low complication rate, shorter median hospital stay, and lower cost of care.[40–42] EMR is usually performed using 1 of 2 techniques—with suction (suck-and-cut) or without (lift-and-cut)—using a submucosal injection to separate the mucosa and muscularis propria to reduce the risk of perforation. Normal saline, hypertonic saline, 50% dextrose, 10% glycerol, 5% fructose, fibrinogen mixture, autologous blood, sodium hyaluronate, and hydroxypropyl methylcellulose have been used for injection.[43–47] Nonlifting or puckering of the lesion during injection suggests invasion of the deep submucosa or muscularis propria.

Box 2
Historic JGES criteria for EMR

- Protruded type lesions ≤2 cm
- Flat or depressed lesions ≤1 cm
- Cancers that are limited to the mucosa

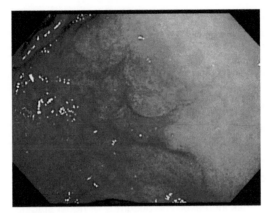

Fig. 1. Well-differentiated EGC in the antrum.

Endoscopic submucosal dissection

Endoscopic submucosal dissection (ESD) was developed in late 1990 to completely remove the gastric dysplasia and cancer regardless of size and location. The size limitation and margin evaluation had been challenges with EMR for gastric cancer in achieving curative resection, especially when it required piecemeal resection. These limitations had caused high rates of residual disease and recurrence, resulting in inferiority to surgical therapy.[48,49] ESD uses a specialized needle knife or equipment to dissect the lesions from the intestinal wall, assisted by a long-lasting submucosal fluid cushion (**Figs. 1–8**).[35,50–53] The major advantage of ESD is that it offers significantly larger en bloc resection of tumor than EMR. It was most extensively investigated for a treatment of EGC,[35,50,54,55] and its use has expanded to lesions in the esophagus and colon.[51,56,57] ESD uses various types of endoscopic electrosurgical needle knives, and many new devices have been developed with improved features for ease and safety. This technique requires advanced skill and training, and is not widely available in the United States except in specialized centers. Details of the ESD procedure are published elsewhere and are beyond the scope of this section.

Meta-analysis of comparative studies of ESD and EMR showed that patients with EGC who underwent ESD had lower rates of local recurrence and higher en bloc

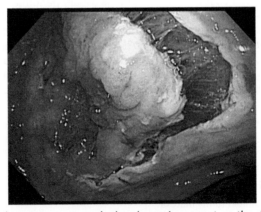

Fig. 2. Borders of the tumor were marked and margin was cut on the right.

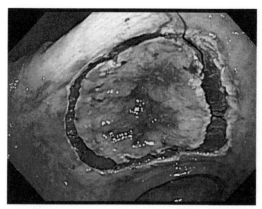

Fig. 3. Circumferential incision of the periphery of the tumor has completed.

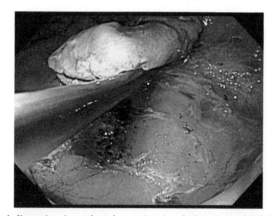

Fig. 4. Submucosal dissection is undertaken using insulation-tipped (IT) knife.

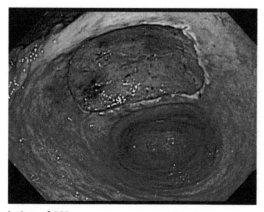

Fig. 5. At the completion of ESD.

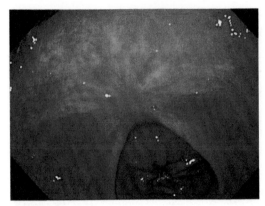

Fig. 6. Healed scar of ESD site.

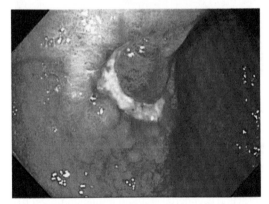

Fig. 7. Large poorly differentiated tumor with ulceration and induration; unsuitable for ESD.

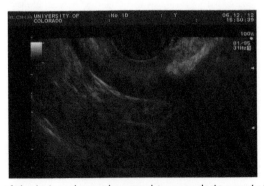

Fig. 8. EUS image of the lesion; deep submucosal to muscularis propria invasion is seen.

and curative resection rates compared with those who underwent EMR for malignant and premalignant lesions of the gastrointestinal tract.[58–60] However, tumors smaller than 10 mm (especially <7 mm) may be managed with EMR with comparable outcome.[55,61,62] The drawbacks of ESD are the longer procedure time and higher risk for intraoperative (but not delayed) bleeding and perforation, although these complications can be managed endoscopically without surgery.[63–65] According to meta-analyses,[59,60,66,67] the perforation rate for ESD was 4.5%, compared with 1.0% for EMR. The factors associated with perforations during ESD were suggested to be tumors of the upper stomach and tumor size greater than 20 mm.[68]

Surgical Resection

Because of the lack of expertise in endoscopic resection techniques, gastrectomy remains the most widely used approach to treating EGC worldwide. Gastrectomy with regional lymph node dissection is recommended for patients who do not fulfill the criteria for endoscopic resection, for whom lymph node metastasis is highly suspected during preoperative staging, or who are at increased risk of lymph node metastases according to postendoscopic resection assessment. Surgical resection for EGC offers a 5-year survival rate of up to 98%. Recurrence rates and mortality after surgery are higher in Western countries[69] than in Asia,[37,66] which may reflect differences in follow-up protocol (endoscopic surveillance for synchronous and metachronous lesions); the extent and method of lymph node dissection (for example, one based on anatomical lymph node distribution for determining accurate stage-specific survival in Asia,[70] and the other in the West based on an absolute number of lymph nodes investigated[71]; and the pathologic criteria used to determine malignancy.

Surveillance for Metachronous Gastric Cancer

Surveillance after treatment of gastric cancer requires special attention. Even though the overall 5-year survival rate for surgically or endoscopically treated EGC is more than 90%,[6,72–74] the recurrence rate is reported from 2 to 15 %, with the higher range quoted in the Western literature.[41,69,75] Regardless of surgical or endoscopic treatment, synchronous and metachronous gastric cancers are seen in patients with EGC.[76–78] High-risk groups for metachronous cancers include patients with multifocal synchronous EGCs, older age, male sex, submucosal invasion, and proximal gastrectomy.[79] Long-term follow-up studies have found that metachronous lesions occur in anywhere from 2% to 8% of patients, including in the gastric remnant, which is seen even after 10 years of surgery.[80–83] While CT scanning, positron emission tomography scanning, and tumor markers are important to detect metastatic recurrence, they play no role in detecting gastric metachronous lesions. Therefore, endoscopic surveillance is advocated for early detection because the survival rate of patients treated for remnant gastric cancer had been low because of discovery at later stage.[75,81,83,84] Endoscopic resection has been applied to metachronous cancer in the gastric remnant and after endoscopic resection and seems to be feasible and safe.[75,78,80,83]

Treatment for Helicobacter pylori Infection

Helicobacter pylori infection is a well-defined risk factor for gastric adenocarcinoma, and chronic infection is associated with metachronous tumors. Treatment of *H pylori* infection has been shown to decrease the risk of developing gastric and metachronous cancer,[85–87] although a longer follow-up period (>5 years) was reported to be associated with less difference in incidence once gastric mucosal atrophy had developed.[88] Based on the available data[87] from a randomized controlled trial, all patients with EGC should be treated for *H pylori* infection if present, and successful eradication should be confirmed with an appropriate test.

INVESTIGATIONS WITH ENDOLUMINAL THERAPY
Standard and Expanding Criteria for Endoscopic Resection, and Risk Stratification

Criteria for selecting appropriate patients with EGC for endoscopic resection with either EMR or ESD are shown in **Box 3**.[4,89] ESD virtually eliminated the restriction on the size of lesion to be removed endoscopically and enabled comprehensive histologic assessment. Gotoda and colleagues[27] proposed a lower-risk category, derived from an analysis of more than 5000 surgical specimens, which allowed the criteria for endoscopic resection to be expanded to larger tumors and an inclusion of certain submucosal tumors (**Box 4**). Submucosal cancer, when it satisfies certain criteria, shows very small risk for lymph node metastasis, similar to mucosal cancer (eg, <30 mm, tumor confined to the upper 0.5 mm of submucosa, absence of lymphovascular invasion), and patients may be followed closely without surgery.[27,90–92] As a result, the traditional consensus indications for gastrectomy with removal of perigastric lymph nodes (**Box 5**) are no longer absolute, and treatment decisions are made based on the availability of endoscopic expertise, comorbidities, and patient preference, especially when presented with the option of minimally invasive surgery.

Curative resection for EGC with ESD

Many retrospective studies[49,93–99] in single and multiple centers evaluated curative resection after ESD. Noncurative resection is defined as the presence of positive lateral or vertical margins, submucosal and lymphovascular invasion, or undifferentiated histology, which implies a higher risk for adverse events (eg, lymph node and distant metastasis or recurrence), and additional surgical therapy is likely beneficial. However, when only positive or unclear lateral margins are seen, this indicates a lower risk for lymph node metastasis in the absence of other factors listed earlier.[100,101] Invasion depth was also carefully evaluated. When the tumor is differentiated and has no lymphovascular invasion, less than 0.5 mm of submucosal involvement is considered a criterion for expanded curative resection.[27] The likelihood of noncurative resection increases with large (>30 mm), piecemeal excised/non–en bloc resected, ulcerated, undifferentiated (especially >20 mm), and deep submucosal (>0.5 mm) tumors; with tumors located in the upper third of the stomach location (for ulcerative tumors in the upper and mid-stomach); and in elderly patients (>75 years of age).[49,93–97] Complication rates of bleeding and perforation associated with ESD may increase based on the expanded criteria compared with the traditional criteria.[98] In elderly patients, ESD

Box 3
Standard criteria for endoscopic resection

1. High probability of en bloc resection
2. Tumor histology
   a. Intestinal-type adenocarcinoma
   b. Tumor confined to the mucosa
3. Tumor size and morphology
   a. Less than 20 mm without ulceration
   b. Less than 10 mm if Paris classification IIb or IIc

> **Box 4**
> **Proposed expanded criteria for endoscopic resection**
>
> 1. Mucosal tumors of any size without ulceration
> 2. Mucosal tumors less than 30 mm with ulceration (1.2 are for differentiated adenocarcinoma)
> 3. Poorly differentiated adenocarcinoma or signet-ring cell carcinoma: Mucosal tumors less than 20 mm without ulceration

remains a valid method for curative resection and should not be excluded, although increased rates of postprocedure pneumonia have been reported.[99]

Management of Incomplete Resection: Piecemeal Versus En Bloc; Positive Margins; and Histologic Risk Factors

In patients with positive lateral margins without other risk factors found on histopathologic evaluation of lesions treated with EMR/ESD, either careful endoscopic follow-up and as-needed adjunct endoscopic therapy or minimally invasive surgery can be considered, because they have a lower risk for experiencing metastasis.[102,103] However, gastrectomy is recommended for patients with positive vertical margins, submucosal involvement (with high-risk features), or lymphovascular invasion.[102,103] Current research focuses on whether patients with incomplete resection after EMR/ESD can be managed with laparoscopic gastrectomy, or even laparoscopic lymph node dissection without gastrectomy when margins are negative.

Laparoscopic gastrectomy
Laparoscopic gastrectomy has been performed in specialized centers. Comparing the outcome with traditional open surgery, laparoscopic approach was shown to benefit patients with lower complications, faster recovery, and improved quality of life.[104–106] Various laparoscopic surgical techniques are being implemented based on location (distal versus proximal), tumor characteristics, and the field of lymph node dissection.

Laparoscopic lymph node dissection without gastrectomy
Another area of active investigation is laparoscopic lymph node dissection without gastrectomy in patients treated with ESD who have negative margins but are considered to have had noncurative resections based on the presence of other criteria (ie, submucosal invasion, lymphovascular invasion, or undifferentiated adenocarcinoma). The area chosen for lymph node dissection in the small case series was based on the location of the tumor and/or the lymphatic drainage of the stomach visualized with standard laparoscopy or infrared-ray electronic laparoscopy after submucosal injection of indocyanine green (ICG) around post-ESD scars (sentinel lymph node). A retrospective study of 21 patients showed that 10% (n = 2) had lymph node metastases confirmed after lymph node dissection without gastrectomy, and none had local or

> **Box 5**
> **Indication for gastrectomy with removal of perigastric lymph nodes**
>
> 1. Low probability of en bloc resection with EMR or ESD, most likely piecemeal
> 2. Diffuse-type (undifferentiated) adenocarcinoma
> 3. Submucosal tumor size greater than 30 mm, or tumors with ulceration
> 4. Evidence of lymphovascular invasion in the primary tumor, or known/suspected lymph node metastasis

distant recurrence at a median follow-up of 61 months.[107] This approach may be acceptable for carefully selected patients. Further prospective comparison studies are needed to generalize this approach to clinical practice.

ONGOING CLINICAL INVESTIGATIONS
Poorly Differentiated Adenocarcinoma

Traditionally, poorly differentiated adenocarcinomas (including signet ring cell carcinoma and mucinous adenocarcinoma) were not considered candidates for endoscopic resection. Therefore, endoscopic management is controversial, and lacks well-designed controlled prospective studies. However, small studies have shown success with endoscopic resection (ESD) for lesions smaller than 20 mm with no lymphovascular invasion.[108,109] For larger-sized lesions showing submucosal invasion and ulceration (reported risk factors for incomplete resection), curative resection with ESD is less possible, and traditional surgery or salvage gastrectomy with lymph node dissection is recommended.[110]

Sentinel Lymph Node Navigation, Mapping, and Biopsy

As the indications for endoscopic resection expand, the issue of possible lymph node involvement will be encountered more frequently after pathologic evaluation on resected specimens. The decision to recommend traditional radical lymphadenectomy may be guided by further limited sampling of lymph node. The sentinel lymph node is the first lymph node that receives lymphatic drainage from the primary tumor site and can be considered the first site of micrometastasis along the route of lymphatic drainage. Studies are investigating sentinel lymph node mapping and navigation using radiocolloid dye or ICG injected endoscopically,[111–114] or CT lymphography using nanoscale iodized oil emulsion[115] to increase the accuracy of detecting lymph node metastasis.[116]

Endoscopic Full-Thickness Resection/Laparoscopic Intragastric Full-Thickness Excision

The indication for this new method is limited because of the potential for tumor dissemination into the abdominal space during the procedure. However, techniques are being developed to accomplish nonexposed endoscopic wall–inversion surgery, which may be an alternative to surgery in patients with submucosal tumor with or without ulceration, or mucosal tumors technically difficult to resect with ESD.[117–119]

FUTURE DIRECTIONS

With the advancement of equipment, techniques, and training, EMR and ESD will become the mainstay of treatment of EGC worldwide. Surgical therapy is also evolving as a primary and salvage treatment and is still a standard treatment for certain patients. Early detection of gastric neoplasia is the key to improving outcomes of patients with gastric cancer. Several areas for future development are worth mentioning.

Improving Detection

Improvement in detection and evaluation of EGC continues to be a focus of research. Autofluorescence imaging (AFI) achieved increased sensitivity but it has a high false-positive rate. Magnifying chromoendoscopy (ie, NBI) and confocal laser endomicroscopy (CLE) have been shown to increase sensitivity and specificity compared with conventional white light endoscopy (c-WLE). Magnifying NBI combined with c-WLE showed excellent detection rates, better than either technique alone. However, the superiority of these techniques seems to depend on local expertise. Although it may show comparable categorical accuracy compared with histologic assessment, CLE is time-consuming and costly, and has a limited role in primary diagnosis and staging.[23,120,121] Trimodal imaging combining c-WLE, NBI, and AFI showed higher sensitivity and specificity.[122] Nevertheless, no established advanced-imaging technique currently exists that is effective for common clinical use.

Robotic Surgery

A comparative study between robotic and laparoscopic radical gastrectomy and other small trials have reported better short-term oncologic outcomes with robotic surgery.[123–125] Robotic surgery can incorporate sentinel lymph node mapping or navigation. It must be compared with combined ESD and laparoscopic lymph node surgery for EGC that is borderline or unsuitable for sole endoscopic treatment.

Molecular Techniques

Several studies have examined microsatellite instability and various oncogenes in endoscopically resected specimens for predicting lymph node metastasis and recurrence, especially in metachronous cancers.[126–128] Several molecular approaches are also being incorporated in sentinel lymph node mapping techniques. The use of quantitative multimarker real-time reverse transcription–polymerase chain reaction was reported for detecting a micrometastasis that may not have been detected histopathologically.[129]

REFERENCES

1. Ferlay J, Shin HR, Bray F, et al. Estimates of worldwide burden of cancer in 2008: GLOBOCAN 2008. Int J Cancer 2010;127(12):2893–917.
2. Jemal A, Siegel R, Xu J, et al. Cancer statistics, 2010. CA Cancer J Clin 2010; 60(5):277–300.
3. Alfaro EE, Lauwers GY. Early gastric neoplasia: diagnosis and implications. Adv Anat Pathol 2011;18(4):268–80.
4. Gotoda T. Endoscopic resection of early gastric cancer: the Japanese perspective. Curr Opin Gastroenterol 2006;22(5):561–9.
5. Shimizu S, Tada M, Kawai K. Early gastric cancer: its surveillance and natural course. Endoscopy 1995;27(1):27–31.
6. Maehara Y, Orita H, Okuyama T, et al. Predictors of lymph node metastasis in early gastric cancer. Br J Surg 1992;79(3):245–7.
7. Noguchi Y, Yoshikawa T, Tsuburaya A, et al. Is gastric carcinoma different between Japan and the United States? Cancer 2000;89(11):2237–46.
8. Schlemper RJ, Riddell RH, Kato Y, et al. The Vienna classification of gastrointestinal epithelial neoplasia. Gut 2000;47(2):251–5.
9. Japanese Gastric Cancer Association. Japanese classification of gastric carcinoma - 3rd English edition. Gastric Cancer 2011;14:101–12.
10. The Paris endoscopic classification of superficial neoplastic lesions: esophagus, stomach, and colon: November 30 to December 1, 2002. Gastrointest Endosc 2003;58(Suppl 6):S3–43.
11. Nishida T, Tsutsui S, Kato M, et al. Treatment strategy for gastric non-invasive intraepithelial neoplasia diagnosed by endoscopic biopsy. World J Gastrointest Pathophysiol 2011;2(6):93–9.
12. Park SY, Jeon SW, Jung MK, et al. Long-term follow-up study of gastric intraepithelial neoplasias: progression from low-grade dysplasia to invasive carcinoma. Eur J Gastroenterol Hepatol 2008;20(10):966–70.

13. Yamada H, Ikegami M, Shimoda T, et al. Long-term follow-up study of gastric adenoma/dysplasia. Endoscopy 2004;36(5):390–6.
14. Bearzi I, Brancorsini D, Santinelli A, et al. Gastric dysplasia: a ten-year follow-up study. Pathol Res Pract 1994;190(1):61–8.
15. Ang TL, Khor CJ, Gotoda T. Diagnosis and endoscopic resection of early gastric cancer. Singapore Med J 2010;51(2):93–100.
16. Kajitani T. The general rules for the gastric cancer study in surgery and pathology. Part I. Clinical classification. Jpn J Surg 1981;11(2):127–39.
17. Lee BE, Kim GH, Park do Y, et al. Acetic acid-indigo carmine chromoendoscopy for delineating early gastric cancers: its usefulness according to histological type. BMC Gastroenterol 2010;10:97.
18. Iizuka T, Kikuchi D, Hoteya S, et al. The acetic acid + indigocarmine method in the delineation of gastric cancer. J Gastroenterol Hepatol 2008;23(9):1358–61.
19. Kuznetsov K, Lambert R, Rey JF. Narrow-band imaging: potential and limitations. Endoscopy 2006;38(1):76–81.
20. Muto M, Katada C, Sano Y, et al. Narrow band imaging: a new diagnostic approach to visualize angiogenesis in superficial neoplasia. Clin Gastroenterol Hepatol 2005;3(7 Suppl 1):S16–20.
21. Kato M, Kaise M, Yonezawa J, et al. Magnifying endoscopy with narrow-band imaging achieves superior accuracy in the differential diagnosis of superficial gastric lesions identified with white-light endoscopy: a prospective study. Gastrointest Endosc 2010;72(3):523–9.
22. Tada K, Oda I, Yokoi C, et al. Pilot study on clinical effectiveness of autofluorescence imaging for early gastric cancer diagnosis by less experienced endoscopists. Diagn Ther Endosc 2011;2011:419136.
23. Ezoe Y, Muto M, Uedo N, et al. Magnifying narrowband imaging is more accurate than conventional white-light imaging in diagnosis of gastric mucosal cancer. Gastroenterology 2011;141(6):2017–2025.e3.
24. Chai NL, Ling-Hu EQ, Morita Y, et al. Magnifying endoscopy in upper gastroenterology for assessing lesions before completing endoscopic removal. World J Gastroenterol 2012;18(12):1295–307.
25. Choi J, Kim SG, Im JP, et al. Endoscopic prediction of tumor invasion depth in early gastric cancer. Gastrointest Endosc 2011;73(5):917–27.
26. Roviello F, Rossi S, Marrelli D, et al. Number of lymph node metastases and its prognostic significance in early gastric cancer: a multicenter Italian study. J Surg Oncol 2006;94(4):275–80 [discussion: 274].
27. Gotoda T, Yanagisawa A, Sasako M, et al. Incidence of lymph node metastasis from early gastric cancer: estimation with a large number of cases at two large centers. Gastric Cancer 2000;3(4):219–25.
28. Nasu J, Nishina T, Hirasaki S, et al. Predictive factors of lymph node metastasis in patients with undifferentiated early gastric cancers. J Clin Gastroenterol 2006;40(5):412–5.
29. Sano T, Kobori O, Muto T. Lymph node metastasis from early gastric cancer: endoscopic resection of tumour. Br J Surg 1992;79(3):241–4.
30. An JY, Baik YH, Choi MG, et al. Predictive factors for lymph node metastasis in early gastric cancer with submucosal invasion: analysis of a single institutional experience. Ann Surg 2007;246(5):749–53.
31. Yoshida S, Tanaka S, Kunihiro K, et al. Diagnostic ability of high-frequency ultrasound probe sonography in staging early gastric cancer, especially for submucosal invasion. Abdom Imaging 2005;30(5):518–23.

32. Yanai H, Fujimura H, Suzumi M, et al. Delineation of the gastric muscularis mucosae and assessment of depth of invasion of early gastric cancer using a 20-megahertz endoscopic ultrasound probe. Gastrointest Endosc 1993;39(4):505–12.

33. Yanai H, Tada M, Karita M, et al. Diagnostic utility of 20-megahertz linear endoscopic ultrasonography in early gastric cancer. Gastrointest Endosc 1996;44(1): 29–33.

34. Kim JH, Song KS, Youn YH, et al. Clinicopathologic factors influence accurate endosonographic assessment for early gastric cancer. Gastrointest Endosc 2007;66(5):901–8.

35. Gotoda T, Yamamoto H, Soetikno RM. Endoscopic submucosal dissection of early gastric cancer. J Gastroenterol 2006;41(10):929–42.

36. Takekoshi T, Baba Y, Ota H, et al. Endoscopic resection of early gastric carcinoma: results of a retrospective analysis of 308 cases. Endoscopy 1994; 26(4):352–8.

37. Raju GS, Waxman I. High-frequency US probe sonography-assisted endoscopic mucosal resection. Gastrointest Endosc 2000;52(Suppl 6):S39–49.

38. Schlemper RJ, Itabashi M, Kato Y, et al. Differences in diagnostic criteria for gastric carcinoma between Japanese and western pathologists. Lancet 1997; 349(9067):1725–9.

39. Kojima T, Parra-Blanco A, Takahashi H, et al. Outcome of endoscopic mucosal resection for early gastric cancer: review of the Japanese literature. Gastrointest Endosc 1998;48(5):550–4 [discussion: 554–5].

40. Uedo N, Iishi H, Tatsuta M, et al. Longterm outcomes after endoscopic mucosal resection for early gastric cancer. Gastric Cancer 2006;9(2):88–92.

41. Hiki Y, Shimao H, Mieno H, et al. Modified treatment of early gastric cancer: evaluation of endoscopic treatment of early gastric cancers with respect to treatment indication groups. World J Surg 1995;19(4):517–22.

42. Manner H, Rabenstein T, May A, et al. Long-term results of endoscopic resection in early gastric cancer: the Western experience. Am J Gastroenterol 2009;104(3):566–73.

43. Sato T. A novel method of endoscopic mucosal resection assisted by submucosal injection of autologous blood (blood patch EMR). Dis Colon Rectum 2006;49(10):1636–41.

44. Fujishiro M, Yahagi N, Kashimura K, et al. Different mixtures of sodium hyaluronate and their ability to create submucosal fluid cushions for endoscopic mucosal resection. Endoscopy 2004;36(7):584–9.

45. Fujishiro M, Yahagi N, Kashimura K, et al. Comparison of various submucosal injection solutions for maintaining mucosal elevation during endoscopic mucosal resection. Endoscopy 2004;36(7):579–83.

46. Lee SH, Park JH, Park do H, et al. Clinical efficacy of EMR with submucosal injection of a fibrinogen mixture: a prospective randomized trial. Gastrointest Endosc 2006;64(5):691–6.

47. Yamamoto H, Yahagi N, Oyama T, et al. Usefulness and safety of 0.4% sodium hyaluronate solution as a submucosal fluid "cushion" in endoscopic resection for gastric neoplasms: a prospective multicenter trial. Gastrointest Endosc 2008;67(6):830–9.

48. Horiki N, Omata F, Uemura M, et al. Risk for local recurrence of early gastric cancer treated with piecemeal endoscopic mucosal resection during a 10-year follow-up period. Surg Endosc 2012;26(1):72–8.

49. Isomoto H, Shikuwa S, Yamaguchi N, et al. Endoscopic submucosal dissection for early gastric cancer: a large-scale feasibility study. Gut 2009;58(3):331–6.

50. Ono H. Endoscopic submucosal dissection for early gastric cancer. Chin J Dig Dis 2005;6(3):119–21.
51. Yamamoto H, Yahagi N, Oyama T. Mucosectomy in the colon with endoscopic submucosal dissection. Endoscopy 2005;37(8):764–8.
52. Oyama T, Tomori A, Hotta K, et al. Endoscopic submucosal dissection of early esophageal cancer. Clin Gastroenterol Hepatol 2005;3(7 Suppl 1):S67–70.
53. Fujishiro M, Yahagi N, Nakamura M, et al. Successful outcomes of a novel endoscopic treatment for GI tumors: endoscopic submucosal dissection with a mixture of high-molecular-weight hyaluronic acid, glycerin, and sugar. Gastrointest Endosc 2006;63(2):243–9.
54. Kim JH, Lee YC, Kim H, et al. Endoscopic resection for undifferentiated early gastric cancer. Gastrointest Endosc 2009;69(4):e1–9.
55. Nakamoto S, Sakai Y, Kasanuki J, et al. Indications for the use of endoscopic mucosal resection for early gastric cancer in Japan: a comparative study with endoscopic submucosal dissection. Endoscopy 2009;41(9):746–50.
56. Fujishiro M, Yahagi N, Kakushima N, et al. Outcomes of endoscopic submucosal dissection for colorectal epithelial neoplasms in 200 consecutive cases. Clin Gastroenterol Hepatol 2007;5(6):678–83 [quiz: 645].
57. Byeon JS, Yang DH, Kim KJ, et al. Endoscopic submucosal dissection with or without snaring for colorectal neoplasms. Gastrointest Endosc 2011;74(5): 1075–83.
58. Cao Y, Liao C, Tan A, et al. Meta-analysis of endoscopic submucosal dissection versus endoscopic mucosal resection for tumors of the gastrointestinal tract. Endoscopy 2009;41(9):751–7.
59. Park YM, Cho E, Kang HY, et al. The effectiveness and safety of endoscopic submucosal dissection compared with endoscopic mucosal resection for early gastric cancer: a systematic review and metaanalysis. Surg Endosc 2011;25(8): 2666–77.
60. Lian J, Chen S, Zhang Y, et al. A meta-analysis of endoscopic submucosal dissection and EMR for early gastric cancer. Gastrointest Endosc 2012;76(4): 763–70.
61. Watanabe T, Kume K, Taip M, et al. Gastric mucosal cancer smaller than 7 mm can be treated with conventional endoscopic mucosal resection as effectively as with endoscopic submucosal dissection. Hepatogastroenterology 2010; 57(99–100):668–73.
62. Watanabe K, Ogata S, Kawazoe S, et al. Clinical outcomes of EMR for gastric tumors: historical pilot evaluation between endoscopic submucosal dissection and conventional mucosal resection. Gastrointest Endosc 2006; 63(6):776–82.
63. Gotoda T. Endoscopic resection of early gastric cancer. Gastric Cancer 2007; 10(1):1–11.
64. Minami S, Gotoda T, Ono H, et al. Complete endoscopic closure of gastric perforation induced by endoscopic resection of early gastric cancer using endoclips can prevent surgery (with video). Gastrointest Endosc 2006;63(4): 596–601.
65. Tsunada S, Ogata S, Ohyama T, et al. Endoscopic closure of perforations caused by EMR in the stomach by application of metallic clips. Gastrointest Endosc 2003;57(7):948–51.
66. Park JC, Lee SK, Seo JH, et al. Predictive factors for local recurrence after endoscopic resection for early gastric cancer: long-term clinical outcome in a single-center experience. Surg Endosc 2010;24(11):2842–9.

67. Takahashi H, Arimura Y, Masao H, et al. Endoscopic submucosal dissection is superior to conventional endoscopic resection as a curative treatment for early squamous cell carcinoma of the esophagus (with video). Gastrointest Endosc 2010;72(2):255–64, 264.e1-2.
68. Ohta T, Ishihara R, Uedo N, et al. Factors predicting perforation during endoscopic submucosal dissection for gastric cancer. Gastrointest Endosc 2012; 75(6):1159–65.
69. Percivale P, Bertoglio S, Muggianu M, et al. Long-term postoperative results in 54 cases of early gastric cancer: the choice of surgical procedure. Eur J Surg Oncol 1989;15(5):436–40.
70. Bunt AM, Hermans J, Smit VT, et al. Surgical/pathologic-stage migration confounds comparisons of gastric cancer survival rates between Japan and Western countries. J Clin Oncol 1995;13(1):19–25.
71. Smith DD, Schwarz RR, Schwarz RE. Impact of total lymph node count on staging and survival after gastrectomy for gastric cancer: data from a large US-population database. J Clin Oncol 2005;23(28):7114–24.
72. Everett SM, Axon AT. Early gastric cancer in Europe. Gut 1997;41(2):142–50.
73. Yasuda K, Shiraishi N, Suematsu T, et al. Rate of detection of lymph node metastasis is correlated with the depth of submucosal invasion in early stage gastric carcinoma. Cancer 1999;85(10):2119–23.
74. Okada K, Fujisaki J, Yoshida T, et al. Long-term outcomes of endoscopic submucosal dissection for undifferentiated-type early gastric cancer. Endoscopy 2012;44(2):122–7.
75. Youn HG, An JY, Choi MG, et al. Recurrence after curative resection of early gastric cancer. Ann Surg Oncol 2010;17(2):448–54.
76. Etoh T, Katai H, Fukagawa T, et al. Treatment of early gastric cancer in the elderly patient: results of EMR and gastrectomy at a national referral center in Japan. Gastrointest Endosc 2005;62(6):868–71.
77. Choi KS, Jung HY, Choi KD, et al. EMR versus gastrectomy for intramucosal gastric cancer: comparison of long-term outcomes. Gastrointest Endosc 2011;73(5):942–8.
78. Kato M, Nishida T, Yamamoto K, et al. Scheduled endoscopic surveillance controls secondary cancer after curative endoscopic resection for early gastric cancer: a multicentre retrospective cohort study by Osaka University ESD study group. Gut 2012. [Epub ahead of print].
79. Nozaki I, Nasu J, Kubo Y, et al. Risk factors for metachronous gastric cancer in the remnant stomach after early cancer surgery. World J Surg 2010;34(7): 1548–54.
80. Nakajima T, Oda I, Gotoda T, et al. Metachronous gastric cancers after endoscopic resection: how effective is annual endoscopic surveillance? Gastric Cancer 2006;9(2):93–8.
81. Sano T, Sasako M, Kinoshita T, et al. Recurrence of early gastric cancer. Follow-up of 1475 patients and review of the Japanese literature. Cancer 1993;72(11): 3174–8.
82. Seto Y, Nagawa H, Muto T. Impact of lymph node metastasis on survival with early gastric cancer. World J Surg 1997;21(2):186–9 [discussion: 190].
83. Takeda J, Toyonaga A, Koufuji K, et al. Early gastric cancer in the remnant stomach. Hepatogastroenterology 1998;45(23):1907–11.
84. Komatsu S, Ichikawa D, Okamoto K. Progression of remnant gastric cancer is associated with duration of follow-up following distal gastrectomy. World J Gastroenterol 2012;18(22):2832–6.

85. Fuccio L, Zagari RM, Eusebi LH, et al. Meta-analysis: can Helicobacter pylori eradication treatment reduce the risk for gastric cancer? Ann Intern Med 2009;151(2):121–8.

86. Uemura N, Mukai T, Okamoto S, et al. Effect of Helicobacter pylori eradication on subsequent development of cancer after endoscopic resection of early gastric cancer. Cancer Epidemiol Biomarkers Prev 1997;6(8):639–42.

87. Fukase K, Kato M, Kikuchi S, et al. Effect of eradication of Helicobacter pylori on incidence of metachronous gastric carcinoma after endoscopic resection of early gastric cancer: an open-label, randomised controlled trial. Lancet 2008; 372(9636):392–7.

88. Maehata Y, Nakamura S, Fujisawa K, et al. Long-term effect of Helicobacter pylori eradication on the development of metachronous gastric cancer after endoscopic resection of early gastric cancer. Gastrointest Endosc 2012;75(1):39–46.

89. Soetikno R, Kaltenbach T, Yeh R, et al. Endoscopic mucosal resection for early cancers of the upper gastrointestinal tract. J Clin Oncol 2005;23(20):4490–8.

90. Kang HJ, Kim DH, Jeon TY, et al. Lymph node metastasis from intestinal-type early gastric cancer: experience in a single institution and reassessment of the extended criteria for endoscopic submucosal dissection. Gastrointest Endosc 2010;72(3):508–15.

91. Ahn JY, Jung HY, Choi KD, et al. Endoscopic and oncologic outcomes after endoscopic resection for early gastric cancer: 1370 cases of absolute and extended indications. Gastrointest Endosc 2011;74(3):485–93.

92. Jee YS, Hwang SH, Rao J, et al. Safety of extended endoscopic mucosal resection and endoscopic submucosal dissection following the Japanese Gastric Cancer Association treatment guidelines. Br J Surg 2009;96(10):1157–61.

93. Nagano H, Ohyama S, Fukunaga T, et al. Two rare cases of node-positive differentiated gastric cancer despite their infiltration to sm1, their small size, and lack of lymphatic invasion into the submucosal layer. Gastric Cancer 2008;11(1): 53–7 [discussion: 57–8].

94. Yamamoto Y, Fujisaki J, Hirasawa T, et al. Therapeutic outcomes of endoscopic submucosal dissection of undifferentiated-type intramucosal gastric cancer without ulceration and preoperatively diagnosed as 20 millimetres or less in diameter. Dig Endosc 2010;22(2):112–8.

95. Ohnita K, Isomoto H, Yamaguchi N, et al. Factors related to the curability of early gastric cancer with endoscopic submucosal dissection. Surg Endosc 2009; 23(12):2713–9.

96. Hirasawa K, Kokawa A, Oka H, et al. Risk assessment chart for curability of early gastric cancer with endoscopic submucosal dissection. Gastrointest Endosc 2011;74(6):1268–75.

97. Hoteya S, Yamashita S, Kikuchi D, et al. Endoscopic submucosal dissection for submucosal invasive gastric cancer and curability criteria. Dig Endosc 2011; 23(1):30–6.

98. Yamaguchi N, Isomoto H, Fukuda E, et al. Clinical outcomes of endoscopic submucosal dissection for early gastric cancer by indication criteria. Digestion 2009;80(3):173–81.

99. Isomoto H, Ohnita K, Yamaguchi N, et al. Clinical outcomes of endoscopic submucosal dissection in elderly patients with early gastric cancer. Eur J Gastroenterol Hepatol 2010;22(3):311–7.

100. Tokioka S, Umegaki E, Murano M, et al. Utility and problems of endoscopic submucosal dissection for early gastric cancer in elderly patients. J Gastroenterol Hepatol 2012;27(Suppl 3):63–9.

101. Oda I, Gotoda T, Sasako M, et al. Treatment strategy after non-curative endoscopic resection of early gastric cancer. Br J Surg 2008;95(12):1495–500.
102. Nagano H, Ohyama S, Fukunaga T, et al. Indications for gastrectomy after incomplete EMR for early gastric cancer. Gastric Cancer 2005;8(3):149–54.
103. Lee JH, Kim JH, Kim DH, et al. Is surgical treatment necessary after non-curative endoscopic resection for early gastric cancer? J Gastric Cancer 2010;10(4):182–7.
104. Kim YW, Baik YH, Yun YH, et al. Improved quality of life outcomes after laparoscopy-assisted distal gastrectomy for early gastric cancer: results of a prospective randomized clinical trial. Ann Surg 2008;248(5):721–7.
105. Lee JH, Yom CK, Han HS. Comparison of long-term outcomes of laparoscopy-assisted and open distal gastrectomy for early gastric cancer. Surg Endosc 2009;23(8):1759–63.
106. Fujiwara M, Kodera Y, Misawa K, et al. Longterm outcomes of early-stage gastric carcinoma patients treated with laparoscopy-assisted surgery. J Am Coll Surg 2008;206(1):138–43.
107. Abe N, Takeuchi H, Ohki A, et al. Long-term outcomes of combination of endoscopic submucosal dissection and laparoscopic lymph node dissection without gastrectomy for early gastric cancer patients who have a potential risk of lymph node metastasis. Gastrointest Endosc 2011;74(4):792–7.
108. Kamada K, Tomatsuri N, Yoshida N. Endoscopic submucosal dissection for undifferentiated early gastric cancer as the expanded indication lesion. Digestion 2012;85(2):111–5.
109. Kunisaki C, Takahashi M, Nagahori Y, et al. Risk factors for lymph node metastasis in histologically poorly differentiated type early gastric cancer. Endoscopy 2009;41(6):498–503.
110. Goh PG, Jeong HY, Kim MJ, et al. Clinical outcomes of endoscopic submucosal dissection for undifferentiated or submucosal invasive early gastric cancer. Clin Endosc 2011;44(2):116–22.
111. Lips DJ, Schutte HW, van der Linden RL, et al. Sentinel lymph node biopsy to direct treatment in gastric cancer. A systematic review of the literature. Eur J Surg Oncol 2011;37(8):655–61.
112. Morita D, Tsuda H, Ichikura T, et al. Analysis of sentinel node involvement in gastric cancer. Clin Gastroenterol Hepatol 2007;5(9):1046–52.
113. Orsenigo E, Tomajer V, Di Palo S, et al. Sentinel node mapping during laparoscopic distal gastrectomy for gastric cancer. Surg Endosc 2008;22(1):118–21.
114. Kelder W, Nimura H, Takahashi N, et al. Sentinel node mapping with indocyanine green (ICG) and infrared ray detection in early gastric cancer: an accurate method that enables a limited lymphadenectomy. Eur J Surg Oncol 2010;36(6):552–8.
115. Lim JS, Choi J, Song J, et al. Nanoscale iodized oil emulsion: a useful tracer for pretreatment sentinel node detection using CT lymphography in a normal canine gastric model. Surg Endosc 2012;26(8):2267–74.
116. Takeuchi H, Kitagawa Y. New sentinel node mapping technologies for early gastric cancer. Ann Surg Oncol 2012. [Epub ahead of print].
117. Goto O, Mitsui T, Fujishiro M, et al. New method of endoscopic full-thickness resection: a pilot study of non-exposed endoscopic wall-inversion surgery in an ex vivo porcine model. Gastric Cancer 2011;14(2):183–7.
118. Hoya Y, Yamashita M, Sasaki T, et al. Laparoscopic intragastric full-thickness excision (LIFE) of early gastric cancer under flexible endoscopic control–introduction of new technique using animal. Surg Laparosc Endosc Percutan Tech 2007;17(2):111–5.

119. Inoue H, Ikeda H, Hosoya T, et al. Endoscopic mucosal resection, endoscopic submucosal dissection, and beyond: full-layer resection for gastric cancer with nonexposure technique (CLEAN-NET). Surg Oncol Clin N Am 2012;21(1): 129–40.

120. Zhang J, Guo SB, Duan ZJ. Application of magnifying narrow-band imaging endoscopy for diagnosis of early gastric cancer and precancerous lesion. BMC Gastroenterol 2011;11:135.

121. Li WB, Zuo XL, Li CQ, et al. Diagnostic value of confocal laser endomicroscopy for gastric superficial cancerous lesions. Gut 2011;60(3):299–306.

122. Kato M, Kaise M, Yonezawa J, et al. Trimodal imaging endoscopy may improve diagnostic accuracy of early gastric neoplasia: a feasibility study. Gastrointest Endosc 2009;70(5):899–906.

123. Woo Y, Hyung WJ, Pak KH, et al. Robotic gastrectomy as an oncologically sound alternative to laparoscopic resections for the treatment of early-stage gastric cancers. Arch Surg 2011;146(9):1086–92.

124. Eom BW, Yoon HM, Ryu KW, et al. Comparison of surgical performance and short-term clinical outcomes between laparoscopic and robotic surgery in distal gastric cancer. Eur J Surg Oncol 2012;38(1):57–63.

125. Yoon HM, Kim YW, Lee JH, et al. Robot-assisted total gastrectomy is comparable with laparoscopically assisted total gastrectomy for early gastric cancer. Surg Endosc 2012;26(5):1377–81.

126. Kim KM, Kim YS, Cho JY, et al. Significance of microsatellite instability in early gastric cancer treated by endoscopic submucosal dissection. Korean J Gastroenterol 2008;51(3):167–73 [in Korean].

127. Fukuda M, Yokozaki H, Shiba M, et al. Genetic and epigenetic markers to identify high risk patients for multiple early gastric cancers after treatment with endoscopic mucosal resection. J Clin Biochem Nutr 2007;40(3):203–9.

128. Hasuo T, Semba S, Li D, et al. Assessment of microsatellite instability status for the prediction of metachronous recurrence after initial endoscopic submucosal dissection for early gastric cancer. Br J Cancer 2007;96(1):89–94.

129. Takeuchi H, Ueda M, Oyama T, et al. Molecular diagnosis and translymphatic chemotherapy targeting sentinel lymph nodes of patients with early gastrointestinal cancers. Digestion 2010;82(3):187–91.

Endoscopic Diagnosis and Management of Ampullary Lesions

Ihab I. El Hajj, MD, MPH, Gregory A. Coté, MD, MS*

KEYWORDS

- Papillectomy • Endoscopic retrograde cholangiopancreatography • Endoscopy
- Endoscopic ultrasound • Adenoma

KEY POINTS

- Most (>95%) ampullary lesions are adenomas or adenocarcinomas.
- Ampullary adenomas may arise sporadically or in the setting of a polyposis syndrome (eg, familial adenomatous polyposis).
- Cross-sectional imaging (eg, computed tomography) has poor sensitivity for diagnosing ampullary lesions but is superior to endoscopic modalities for the evaluation of distant metastases in the setting of confirmed malignancy.
- Endoscopic inspection using a side-viewing endoscope with directed biopsies is the most accurate diagnostic test. However, submucosal lesions and early adenocarcinoma (within an adenoma) may be missed.
- Endoscopic ultrasound and endoscopic retrograde cholangiopancreatography are important tools for characterizing submucosal lesions, T staging, and assessment of intraductal (biliary, pancreatic, or both) involvement.
- Ampullary adenomas without intraductal extension or extensive duodenal involvement can be excised via endoscopic papillectomy, which has a more favorable risk profile than surgical approaches.
- Limited data support particular techniques for endoscopic resection of adenomas (eg, electrocautery settings, type of snare, use of pancreatobiliary sphincterotomy).
- The clinician should be familiar with the indications, advantages, and limitations of endoscopic papillectomy in the management of these lesions.

Grant Support: None.
Disclosure: None of the authors have any relevant conflicts of interest to disclose.
Department of Medicine, Division of Gastroenterology & Hepatology, Indiana University School of Medicine, Indianapolis, IN, USA
* Corresponding author. Indianapolis University School of Medicine, University Hospital, 550 North University Boulevard, UH 1634, Indianapolis, IN 46202.
E-mail address: gcote@iupui.edu

Gastrointest Endoscopy Clin N Am 23 (2013) 95–109
http://dx.doi.org/10.1016/j.giec.2012.10.004
1052-5157/13/$ – see front matter © 2013 Elsevier Inc. All rights reserved.

giendo.theclinics.com

INTRODUCTION

Lesions of the ampulla of Vater represent an uncommon group of gastrointestinal malignancies. However, their prognosis can be devastating, so early detection is paramount. Advances in endoscopy, particularly endoscopic retrograde cholangiopancreatography (ERCP) and endoscopic ultrasound (EUS), have significantly impacted the clinical approach to patients with suspected premalignant or malignant lesions of this region. Here, the authors discuss the epidemiology of ampullary adenomas; the role of endoscopy, EUS, and ERCP for the diagnosis and local staging of these lesions; and the current evidence evaluating the diagnostic and therapeutic role of endoscopy in their management.

EPIDEMIOLOGY

Lesions of the ampulla of Vater may be classified as benign, premalignant, and malignant (**Table 1**).[1,2] Because the overwhelming majority (>95%) are either adenomas or adenocarcinomas, this article is primarily devoted to the workup and endoscopic treatment of this subtype. The annual incidence of ampullary lesions in the United States is 3,000, with reported prevalence rates of 0.04%–0.12% in autopsy series.[3,4] Ampullary adenomas may occur sporadically or in the setting of hereditary polyposis syndromes, including familial adenomatous polyposis (FAP) with adenomatous polyposis coli gene mutations. In patients with FAP, ampullary adenomas occur in up to 80% of individuals during their lifetime and progress to malignancy in 4%.[5]

Ampullary adenomas are likely to follow an adenoma-to-carcinoma sequence similar to colorectal adenocarcinoma.[6] Heidecke and colleagues[7] emphasized the correlation between the preoperative dysplasia grade and the malignant transformation rate during follow-up. Therefore, these lesions are considered premalignant, with an incidence of transformation to carcinoma ranging from 25%–85% for sporadic

Table 1		
Differential diagnosis of the prominent ampulla		
Benign	**Premalignant**	**Malignant**
Impacted gallstone	Adenoma • Spontaneous • Associated with a polyposis syndrome (eg, familial adenomatous polyposis)	Adenocarcinoma
Papillitis	Choledochocele (type III choledochal cyst)	Metastatic cancer • Breast • Renal • Melanoma
Hamartoma	Intra-ampullary papillary tubular neoplasm[2]	Intramural tumor • Carcinoid • Stromal tumor • Neuroendocrine tumor
Heterotopic gastric mucosa		
Lipoma		

From El Hajj II, DeWitt JM, Cote GA. Diagnosis and staging of premalignant and early malignant diseases of the gallbladder, bile duct, and ampulla of vater. In: Deutsch J, Banks M, editors. Gastrointestinal endoscopy in the cancer patient. Oxford (United Kingdom): Wiley Inc, 2013; with permission.

adenomas. As with all neoplasms, tumor stage dictates the appropriate therapy. Several classification systems have been proposed (**Table 2**).[8-11]

CLINICAL PRESENTATION AND APPROACH TO THE PATIENT

Patients with ampullary lesions may present with biliary colic, obstructive jaundice, or nonspecific upper abdominal pain with or without fluctuating liver function tests, malaise, and anorexia. However, ampullary lesions often are found incidentally on cross-sectional imaging or during upper endoscopy performed for a different indication. For ampullary adenomas, options include observation with surveillance biopsies or attempts to completely resect the lesion via endoscopy or surgery. Surveillance of an ampullary adenoma in the setting of FAP is reasonable if the lesion is small (<1 cm) and asymptomatic. In patients with ampullary adenocarcinoma, palliative stenting can be performed in individuals who have a short life expectancy.

Table 2
Classification systems for ampullary adenomas and adenocarcinomas

Classification System	Description
TNM[9]	Based on depth of invasion • T0, No evidence of primary tumor • Tis, Carcinoma in situ • T1, Tumor echo limited to the major papilla • T2, Invasion of the duodenal muscularis propria • T3, Invasion of the pancreatic parenchyma • T4, Invasion of peripancreatic soft tissue or adjacent organs or structures • N0, No regional lymph node invasion • N1, Regional lymph node invasion • M0, No evidence of distant metastasis • M1, Evidence of distant metastasis

Vienna[10]	Based on histologic grade
	• Category 1, Negative for neoplasia/dysplasia
	• Category 2, Indefinite for neoplasia/dysplasia
	• Category 3, Noninvasive low-grade neoplasia/dysplasia
	• Category 4, Noninvasive high-grade neoplasia
	  ○ High-grade adenoma/dysplasia
	  ○ Noninvasive carcinoma (carcinoma in situ)
	  ○ Suspicion of invasive carcinoma
	• Category 5, Invasive neoplasia
	  ○ Intramucosal carcinoma
	  ○ Submucosal carcinoma or beyond

Spigelman[11,a]	Based on scoring and staging system, specifically in FAP patients Scoring (1–3 for each variable): • Number of polyps (1–4; 5–20; >20) • Size (1–4; 5–10; >10) • Histologic type (tubular, tubulovillous, villous) • Degree of dysplasia (mild, moderate, and severe) Staging: • Stage I: score 1–4 • Stage II: score 5–6 • Stage III: score 7–8 • Stage IV: score 9–12

[a] Spigelman classification pertains to duodenal pathology (in addition to the ampulla) in patients with FAP.

Historically, surgical resection has been the standard for ampullary resection. Treatment modalities include pancreatoduodenectomy (traditional or pylorus preserving) and transduodenal excision. Pancreatoduodenectomy is associated with higher morbidity (50%–60%) and mortality (0%–9%) compared with transduodenal excision (morbidity, 14%–27%; mortality 0%–4%).[12] However, the largest series of surgical excision of ampullary adenomas and adenocarcinomas reported high recurrence rates (30%) with transduodenal excision, obligating close endoscopic surveillance after surgery.[13]

In patients with ampullary adenomas, endoscopic resection represents an alternative to surgical therapy in appropriately selected patients. Endoscopic papillectomy was first described in 1983 by Suzuki and colleagues[14] and the first large case series described in 1993 by Binmoeller and colleagues.[15] Since, many other series have reported low morbidity and mortality with endoscopic therapy.[16–31]

DIAGNOSIS AND LOCAL STAGING

Cross-sectional imaging, including multidetector computed tomography (MDCT), magnetic resonance imaging, and positron emission tomography (PET), have a low sensitivity for the primary diagnosis of ampullary lesions. Their utility is typically limited to staging of known ampullary cancers. Therefore, endoscopy and endoscopic ultrasound represent the principal modalities for diagnosis.

Endoscopy

Endoscopic inspection with a forward-viewing endoscope is inadequate for distinguishing a prominent but otherwise normal ampulla from alternate etiologies; thus, inspection with a side-viewing endoscope is essential.[32] Endoscopic features of noncancerous lesions include the presence of a regular margin, absence of ulceration or spontaneous bleeding, and having a soft consistency.[16] A principal advantage of side-viewing endoscopy is its ability to easily obtain tissue biopsies at the time of the procedure. Forceps biopsies have high sensitivity (>90%) for confirming the presence of adenoma but lower sensitivity for confirming adenocarcinoma, missing the diagnosis in up to 30% of cases.[33,34] The frequency of malignant foci in ampullary adenomas is reported in the literature at 26%–30%. Therefore, a negative biopsy result does not exclude the presence of cancer, and a minimum of 6 forceps biopsies has been recommended. For this reason, surveillance of sporadic (ie, non-FAP-associated) ampullary adenomas generally is not recommended.

Endoscopic Ultrasound

EUS is consistently more accurate than MDCT, transabdominal ultrasound scan, magnetic resonance imaging, and angiography for T staging of ampullary cancers.[35–38] EUS is a useful adjunct to side-viewing endoscopy to assess for infiltration of the periampullary wall layers, the common bile duct, or ventral pancreatic duct (**Fig. 1**). Specifically, the accuracy of EUS for classifying a cancer as at least a T1 tumor (and thus excluding endoscopic or limited surgical resection) is approximately 90%.[37,38] Most reported discrepancies result from the understaging of T3 and overstaging of T2 lesions, which is unlikely to impact the decision for surgical resection.[39] However, EUS is less accurate than MDCT in the nodal staging of ampullary carcinomas, with estimates of 53%–87%.[36,37,39,40] EUS is also useful for diagnosing nonadenomatous lesions, such as carcinoid tumors of the ampulla. This is germane when forceps biopsies of a prominent ampulla return normal-appearing mucosa.

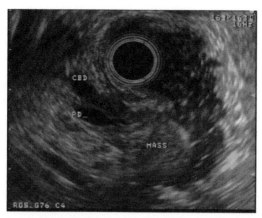

Fig. 1. EUS of ampullary adenoma shows a 23-mm x 20-mm, hypoechoic, well-defined mass in the ampulla. The lesion extends from the mucosa without invasion of the submucosa or muscularis propria. The adjacent pancreatic duct (PD) and common bile duct (CBD) are intact. EUS–fine-needle aspiration confirmed tubular adenoma. (*From* El Hajj II, DeWitt JM, Cote GA. Diagnosis and staging of premalignant and early malignant diseases of the gallbladder, bile duct, and ampulla of vater. In: Deutsch J, Banks M, editors. Gastrointestinal endoscopy in the cancer patient. Oxford (United Kingdom): Wiley Inc, 2013; with permission.)

Several trials have compared standard EUS using radial or linear array echoendoscopes with intraductal ultrasound (IDUS) (**Table 3**).[40–42] In 2 studies, IDUS was superior to EUS in terms of tumor visualization and T staging. However, because of its more cumbersome application and increased risk compared with standard EUS, the clinical utility of IDUS remains unclear. Although EUS may obviate the need for ERCP to evaluate for intraductal extension in some cases, it does not have to be universally incorporated into the diagnostic evaluation of an ampullary adenoma. If the clinical suspicion for invasive carcinoma is low (eg, absence of jaundice and endoscopic features described above), and the lesion appears amenable to endoscopic resection, then EUS may not impact the endoscopist's decision to stage the lesion via papillectomy.

Endoscopic Retrograde Cholangiopancreatography

Tumor involvement of the bile or pancreatic duct significantly reduces the likelihood of complete resection via endoscopic papillectomy. Therefore, ERCP is an important part of the pretreatment staging of ampullary adenomas and for the palliation of obstructive jaundice in the setting of ampullary adenocarcinoma. In the absence of

Table 3		
Diagnostic accuracy of EUS and IDUS for T staging in ampullary cancers		
	Overall Accuracy	
Study	**EUS**	**IDUS**
Itoh et al,[40] 1997	90% (29/32)	88% (28/32)
Menzel et al,[41] 1999	62% (5/8)	93% (14/15)
Ito et al,[42] 2007	63% (25/40)	78% (31/40)

confirmed malignancy, ERCP typically is performed at the time of endoscopic papillectomy to (1) evaluate for intraductal extension and (2) deploy a prophylactic pancreatic duct stent to minimize the risk of post-ERCP pancreatitis after ampullectomy. The
accuracy of ERCP compared with EUS for delineating ductal extension of tumor
requires further study. Therefore, most endoscopists will perform a cholangiopancrea-
togram at the time of resection unless EUS had previously confirmed ductal involvement.[43] In that case, endoscopic resection is usually not attempted. The authors'
practice typically follows a diagnostic and treatment algorithm based on the presence
of adenoma and polyposis syndrome (**Fig. 2**).

ENDOSCOPIC THERAPY

If invasive adenocarcinoma is not identified on forceps biopsies and the adenoma
appears amenable to endoscopic resection after white light endoscopy and cholangiopancreatography, endoscopic papillectomy should be considered in lieu of surgical
resection. Relative exclusion criteria for endoscopic resection include: tumor size
greater than 4 cm, endoscopic findings suspicious for malignancy (ie, indurated or
ulcerated mass), intraductal extension on EUS or ERCP, poor patient compliance
with follow-up, and absence of endoscopic expertise.[15,18,25] However, there are

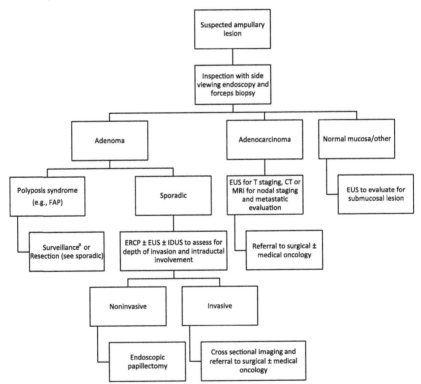

Fig. 2. Recommended algorithm for evaluating a suspected ampullary lesion. [a] Surveillance
of ampullary adenomas in the setting of FAP or other polyposis syndromes is reasonable if
the lesion is small (<1 cm) and the patient is asymptomatic. CT, computed tomography; MRI,
magnetic resonance imaging.

isolated reports of endoscopic resection of large adenomas up to 7 cm,[19] lesions with intraductal growth,[28] and early T1 ampullary adenocarcinoma.[44]

The terms *endoscopic ampullectomy* and *endoscopic papillectomy* are used interchangeably in clinical practice. Technically, *ampullectomy* is defined as circumferential resection of the ampulla of Vater, with separate reinsertion of the common bile duct and the main pancreatic duct into the duodenal wall. Thus, the term *papillectomy* is more appropriate for papillary adenomas removed endoscopically.[45] Papillectomy is one of the more advanced endoscopic maneuvers completed by an interventional endoscopist. It involves techniques of ERCP, tissue resection, hemostasis, and specimen retrieval. Although complex, in skilled hands, the procedure should have a minimally increased risk profile compared with therapeutic ERCP.[25,46] There are variations of the technique that are primarily based on anecdotal experience or personal preference. Limited comparative studies inform an evidence-based approach.

TECHNIQUES OF ENDOSCOPIC PAPILLECTOMY
Submucosal Injection

The role of submucosal injection of saline or diluted epinephrine before ampullectomy is unclear.[25,30] Methylene blue can be added to the saline solution to better visualize the margins of the tumor.[30] The use of a submucosal fluid cushion converts en bloc ampullectomy to a mucosectomy; however, ampullary tumors differ from mucosal neoplasms in that the bile and pancreatic ducts are embedded in the tissue. A mucosal lift hinders access to both bile and pancreatic ducts and interferes with complete resection of ampullary adenomas to the level of the sphincter muscle.[29] Furthermore, injection may create a dome effect and make effective snare placement for en bloc resection more difficult.[47] Finally, there are reports of increased risk of postresection pancreatitis. For these reasons, and the paucity of evidence suggesting it lowers the rate of perforation or hemorrhage, the authors do not perform submucosal injection before papillectomy.

Endoscopic Resection

There is no consensus as to which type of snare should be used for endoscopic papillectomy. Standard braided polypectomy snares typically are used; however, spiral and fine wire snares specifically designed for ampullary resection are available. The diameter of the snare depends on the size of the tumor. The use of electrosurgical needle knife to make an incision circumferentially around the lesion to facilitate snare capture has been reported.[25] There is no evidence to support one type or size of snare over others.

For most ampullary lesions, it is easy to place a standard oval snare tip against the wall of the duodenum at the superior aspect of the mass.[27] As the snare is slowly opened, the endoscope is advanced slightly to allow the snare to open around the entire lesion. The snare is then retracted as the operator advances the snare catheter to the distal base of the lesion, resulting in complete entrapment of the papilla and lesion (**Fig. 3**A,B). The elevator can be lowered and the scope manipulated to assess adequacy of tissue entrapment and to be certain that excessive normal duodenal mucosa has not been incorporated.

En Bloc or Piecemeal Resection

In general, en bloc resection should be attempted in all cases. This method has the advantage of reducing the procedure time and providing clear margins for histopathologic evaluation (see **Fig. 3**C). Piecemeal resection is usually reserved for cases in

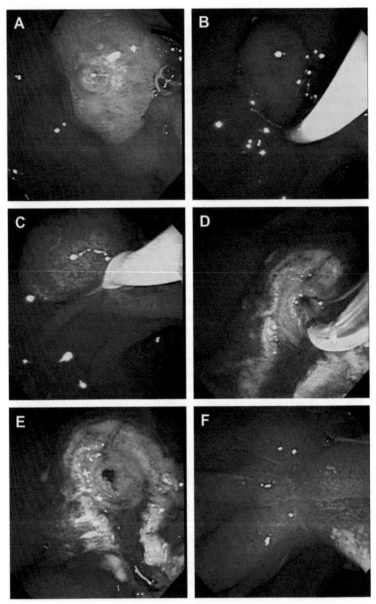

Fig. 3. Endoscopic removal of ampullary adenoma. Endoscopy shows an ampullary adenoma (*A*). The lesion was grasped using a polypectomy snare (*B*). Using a blended elec-trocautery current, the lesion was resected en bloc (*C*). A sphincterotome was used to perform a biliary sphincterotomy (*D*), leaving a patent biliary orifice at the completion of the procedure (*E*). No residual adenoma was identified 3 months later on surveillance endos-copy with biopsies (*F*). (*From* El Hajj II, DeWitt JM, Cote GA. Diagnosis and staging of prema-lignant and early malignant diseases of the gallbladder, bile duct, and ampulla of vater. In: Deutsch J, Banks M, editors. Gastrointestinal endoscopy in the cancer patient. Oxford (United Kingdom): Wiley Inc, 2013; with permission.)

which an attempt at en bloc resection has failed. Some have postulated that this technique decreases recurrence rates, bleeding, and perforation.[18] Comparative trials are lacking; generally speaking, lesions requiring piecemeal resection represent larger or more sessile growths that are more likely to have higher rates of incomplete resection.

Electrocautery Settings

There is no consensus regarding the optimal current (cut, coagulation, or blended) and power output for endoscopic papillectomy. Some studies report using a blended electrosurgical current,[15,25,26] whereas others report using a pure cutting current[15,28,48] or alternating cut/coagulation modes.[25,31,49] One study reported the use of pure coagulation current,[18] although this can cause increased tissue edema at the site of resection. Power output ranges from 30 to 150 W.[18,25,26,48] In general, some cutting current is required to resect the lesion while minimizing the cautery effect at the level of the papilla. A blended or alternating current are advocated by most experts (see **Fig. 3**C).

Tissue Retrieval and Postprocedure Inspection

Recovery of all resected specimens is important for detecting small malignant foci. Small pieces can be aspirated through the scope with a suction trap in place. Rapid entrapment of the en bloc specimen or larger pieces of resected tissue with the snare, retrieval net, or other device is essential to prevent loss of the specimen into the jejunum. During the exchange of accessories, the resected specimen can be held using endoscopic suction to prevent tissue migration. Once retrieved, the specimen can be pinned to a polystyrene block to aid orientation and facilitate margin analysis. The pathology report should document the size, gross appearance, histology, microscopic depth, ductal involvement, specimen integrity (intact, fragmented), and margin status. After specimen retrieval, the duodenoscope should be reintroduced to examine the resection site for active bleeding or bleeding stigmata. These can usually be controlled using standard endoscopic modalities.

Thermal Ablation

For residual polyp tissue, thermal modalities include the neodymium:yttrium-aluminum-garnet laser,[16,26,50] monopolar and bipolar coagulation,[16,18,26,28] and argon plasma coagulation.[3,16,30] There are no randomized, controlled trials comparing individual modalities, and the technical approach depends on availability and preference of the endoscopist. In practice, thermal therapy is used more commonly as adjunctive therapy to treat residual adenomatous tissue remaining after snare resection. The benefits of adjunctive therapy remain controversial. In a large series of 103 patients,[26] the overall success rate for papillectomy was similar in patients who had adjuvant thermal ablation (81%) compared with those who did not (78%). Thermal therapy should not be used for primary resection because occult malignancy could be unrecognized, and the rate of complete ablation is low.

Preresection Sphincterotomy

Pancreatic or biliary sphincterotomy before papillectomy theoretically decreases the risk of tissue injury to the pancreatic and biliary orifices during papillectomy, provides pancreatobiliary drainage after papillectomy, and simplifies postpapillectomy deployment of pancreatic or biliary stents.[18] However, preresection sphincterotomy may interfere with subsequent en bloc resection and will hinder complete histologic evaluation of the resected specimen as a result of thermal injury. Increased risks of bleeding, perforation, and tumor seeding also have been suggested.[51]

Postresection Sphincterotomy and Stent Placement

Careful observation of the resection site usually finds focal orifices representing the insertion of the pancreas and bile ducts into the duodenal wall. To facilitate pancreatic duct cannulation after papillectomy, some endoscopists will perform pancreatography with iodinated contrast diluted with methylene blue before resection. The blue-stained pancreatic orifice can be identified more easily after papillectomy. If prompt cannulation is not obtained, synthetic secretin can be infused to induce juice flow to better identify the orifice and facilitate the cannulation. Anecdotal reports using EUS-directed pancreatography to identify and access the pancreatic duct has been described for particularly difficult cannulation after resection.[52] Postresection pancreatic sphincterotomy probably reduces the incidence of stenosis; furthermore, a pancreatic duct stent should be left in place to reduce the severity and incidence of postpapillectomy pancreatitis.[25,26,29,31]

Attention can then be directed to the biliary orifice (see **Fig. 3E**). Acute cholangitis after endoscopic papillectomy is rare,[53] and prophylactic biliary stent placement is infrequently performed. However, a limited biliary sphincterotomy (see **Fig. 3D**) often is performed to minimize the probability of stenosis despite the absence of comparative trials confirming its benefit.[30]

COMPLICATIONS OF PAPILLECTOMY

Endoscopic papillectomy-related complications in published series are summarized in **Table 4**. Bleeding (0%–25%) and pancreatitis (0%–25%) are seen most frequently. Acute bleeding can usually be managed with typical endoscopic hemostatic techniques. If massive bleeding is encountered, emergent arteriography with embolization typically is preferred to surgical exploration; however, local expertise is best used to dictate the approach in a critically ill patient. Whenever possible, placement of a prophylactic pancreatic duct stent is recommended to reduce the incidence and severity of postpapillectomy pancreatitis.[29,54] Less commonly reported complications include perforation, cholangitis, and stenosis of the pancreatic or biliary orifice. Procedure-related mortality after papillectomy has been reported but is rare, occurring in 2 of 706 reported cases (0.3%).

SURVEILLANCE

In addition to confirming a negative resection margin, histologic review should evaluate for occult adenocarcinoma that could have been missed on forceps biopsies. The presence of in situ carcinoma may impact the surveillance interval, assuming the lesion was completely excised. Adenoma recurrence has been reported in up to 26% of cases despite presumed complete removal during the index procedure.[25,26] In the absence of symptoms, surveillance endoscopy can be accomplished using a side-viewing endoscope without ERCP (see **Fig. 3F**). Intervals vary based on the histology and margin status of the resected lesion, history of FAP, and patient age; if there was no residual polyp after the primary resection, the authors recommend performing a repeat endoscopy 3 months later. If the result is negative for residual adenoma, surveillance 1 year later is probably reasonable. Beyond this, the yield of long-term surveillance in sporadic ampullary adenomas is unknown. Patients with FAP should undergo routine surveillance every 3 years given their risk for metachronous duodenal lesions.

Table 4
Complications related to endoscopic papillectomy in published series

Study	No. of Patients	Bleeding, n (%)	Pancreatitis, n (%)	Perforation	Cholangitis	Stricture	Mortality
Binmoeller et al,[15] 1993	25	2 (8)	3 (12)	0	0	0	0
Martin et al,[16] 1997	14	1 (7)	1 (7)	0	0	0	1
Vogt et al,[17] 2000	18	2 (11)	2 (11)	0	0	0	0
Desilets et al,[18] 2001	13	0	1 (8)	0	0	0	0
Zadorova et al,[19] 2001	16	2 (13)	2 (13)	0	0	0	0
Fukushima et al,[20] 2001	31	4 (13)	4 (13)	0	0	0	0
Norton et al,[21] 2002	26	0	4 (15)	1	0	2	0
Maguchi et al,[22] 2003	12	3 (25)	3 (25)	1	0	0	0
Hirooka et al,[23] 2004	60	8 (13)	6 (10)	0	2	0	0
Han et al,[24] 2004	33	6 (18)	0	1	1	3	0
Cheng et al,[25] 2004	55	4 (7)	5 (9)	1	0	2	0
Catalano et al,[26] 2004	103	2 (2)	5 (5)	0	0	3	0
Kahaleh et al,[27] 2004	56	2 (4)	4 (7)	0	1	0	1
Bohnacker et al,[28] 2005	87	18 (21)	11 (13)	0	0	0	0
Harewood et al,[29] 2005	19	0	3 (16)	0	0	0	0
Irani et al,[30] 2009	102	5 (5)	10 (10)	2	1	3	0
Yamao et al,[31] 2010	36	3 (8)	3 (8)	0	1	0	0
Total (%)	706	62 (9)	67 (9.5)	6 (0.9)	6 (0.9)	13 (1.9)	2 (0.3)

ALTERNATIVE TECHNIQUES

Novel techniques have been proposed, including balloon-catheter–assisted endoscopic snare papillectomy,[48] wire-guided endoscopic snare papillectomy,[55,56] and endoscopic submucosal dissection.[57] The data available on the use of these methods are limited to case reports and small case series. The feasibility and safety of these methods remain to be confirmed at a larger scale.

SUMMARY

Side-viewing endoscopy, EUS, and ERCP are complimentary techniques that have improved diagnostic accuracy and minimized morbidity for the treatment of ampullary lesions. Forceps biopsies of ampullary adenomas have poor sensitivity for confirming the presence of adenocarcinoma, so EUS and ERCP should be considered before proceeding with endoscopic resection in many cases. Endoscopic papillectomy has largely replaced surgical interventions for the treatment of ampullary adenomas without ductal extension. The authors recommend en bloc resection before sphincterotomy whenever possible and performing limited sphincterotomies after resection to minimize the likelihood of pancreatobiliary orifice stenosis later. Future studies should evaluate the impact of EUS/IDUS in predicting complete endoscopic resection and clarify polyp or resection techniques that are associated with higher rates of persistent or recurrent adenoma. Long-term follow-up data are needed to clarify the appropriate surveillance interval for patients with sporadic ampullary adenomas. Collaborative, prospective research among referral centers is necessary, given the low prevalence of ampullary lesions and disparities in resection techniques among expert endoscopists.

REFERENCES

1. El Hajj II, DeWitt JM, Cote GA. Diagnosis and staging of premalignant and early malignant diseases of the gallbladder, bile duct, and ampulla of vater. In: Deutsch J, Banks M, editors. Gastrointestinal endoscopy in the cancer patient. Oxford (United Kingdom): Wiley, Inc, in press.
2. Ohike N, Kim GE, Tajiri T, et al. Intra-ampullary papillary-tubular neoplasm (IAPN): characterization of tumoral intraepithelial neoplasia occurring within the ampulla: a clinicopathologic analysis of 82 cases. Am J Surg Pathol 2010;34:1731–48.
3. Martin JA, Haber GB. Ampullary adenoma: clinical manifestations, diagnosis, and treatment. Gastrointest Endosc Clin N Am 2003;13:649–69.
4. Grobmyer SR, Stasik CN, Draganov P, et al. Contemporary results with ampullectomy for 29 "benign" neoplasms of the ampulla. J Am Coll Surg 2008;206:466–71.
5. Burke CA, Beck GJ, Church JM, et al. The natural history of untreated duodenal and ampullary adenomas in patients with familial adenomatous polyposis followed in an endoscopic surveillance program. Gastrointest Endosc 1999;49: 358–64.
6. Fischer HP, Zhou H. Pathogenesis of carcinoma of the papilla of vater. J Hepatobiliary Pancreat Surg 2004;11:301–9.
7. Heidecke CD, Rosenberg R, Bauer M, et al. Impact of grade of dysplasia in villous adenomas of Vater's papilla. World J Surg 2002;26:709–14.
8. Patel R, Varadajulu S, Wilcox CM. Endoscopic ampullectomy: techniques and outcomes. J Clin Gastroenterol 2012;46:8–15.
9. AJCC Cancer Staging Manual. Exocrine pancreas. American Joint Committee on Cancer Manual. 5th edition. Philadelphia: Lippincott-Raven; 1997. p. 121–6.
10. Schlemper RJ, Riddell RH, Kato Y, et al. The Vienna classification of gastrointestinal epithelial neoplasia. Gut 2000;47:251–5.
11. Spigelman AD, Williams CB, Talbot IC, et al. Upper gastrointestinal cancer in patients with familial adenomatous polyposis. Lancet 1989;2:783–5.
12. de Castro SM, van Heek NT, Kuhlmann KF, et al. Surgical management of neoplasms of the ampulla of Vater: local resection or pancreatoduodenectomy and prognostic factors for survival. Surgery 2004;136:994–1002.

13. Winter JM, Cameron JL, Olino K, et al. Clinicopathologic analysis of ampullary neoplasms in 450 patients: implications for surgical strategy and long-term prognosis. J Gastrointest Surg 2010;14:379–87.
14. Suzuki K, Kantou U, Murakami Y. Two cases with ampullary cancer who underwent endoscopic excision. Prog Dig Endosc 1983;23:236–9.
15. Binmoeller K, Boaventura S, Ramsperger K, et al. Endoscopic snare excision of benign adenomas of the papilla of Vater. Gastrointest Endosc 1993;39:127–31.
16. Martin JA, Haber GB, Kortan PP, et al. Endoscopic snare ampullectomy for resection of benign ampullary neoplasms. Gastrointest Endosc 1997;45(4):AB139.
17. Vogt M, Jakobs R, Benz C, et al. Endoscopic therapy of adenomas of the papilla of Vater. A retrospective analysis with long-term follow-up. Dig Liver Dis 2000;32: 339–45.
18. Desilets DJ, Dy RM, Ku PM, et al. Endoscopic management of tumors of the major duodenal papilla: refined techniques to improve outcome and avoid complications. Gastrointest Endosc 2001;54:202–8.
19. Zadorova Z, Dvorak M, Hajer J. Endoscopic therapy of benign tumors of the papilla of Vater. Endoscopy 2001;33:345–7.
20. Fukushima T, Fogel EL, Devereaux BM, et al. Use of ERCP and papillectomy in management of ampullary tumors: seven-year review of 75 cases at Indiana University Medical Center. Gastrointest Endosc 2001;53:AB88.
21. Norton ID, Gostout CJ, Baron TH, et al. Safety and outcome of endoscopic snare excision of the major duodenal papilla. Gastrointest Endosc 2002;56:239–43.
22. Maguchi H, Takahashi K, Katanuma A, et al. Indication of endoscopic papillectomy for tumors of the papilla of Vater and its problems. Dig Endosc 2003; 15(Suppl):S33–5.
23. Hirooka Y, Itoh A, Goto H. EUS/IDUS and endoscopic papillectomy. Dig Endosc 2004;16:S176–7.
24. Han J, Lee SK, Park DH, et al. Treatment outcome after endoscopic papillectomy of tumors of the major duodenal papilla. Korean J Gastroenterol 2004;29:395.
25. Cheng CL, Sherman S, Fogel EL, et al. Endoscopic snare papillectomy for tumors of the duodenal papillae. Gastrointest Endosc 2004;60:757–64.
26. Catalano MF, Linder JD, Chak A, et al. Endoscopic management of adenoma of the major duodenal papilla. Gastrointest Endosc 2004;59:225–32.
27. Kahaleh M, Shami VM, Brock A, et al. Factors predictive of malignancy and endoscopic resectability in ampullary neoplasia. Am J Gastroenterol 2004;99:2235–9.
28. Bohnacker S, Seitz U, Nguyen D, et al. Endoscopic resection of benign tumors of the duodenal papilla without and with intraductal growth. Gastrointest Endosc 2005;62:551–60.
29. Harewood GC, Pochron NL, Gostout CJ. Prospective, randomized, controlled trial of prophylactic pancreatic stent placement for endoscopic snare excision of the duodenal ampulla. Gastrointest Endosc 2005;62:367–70.
30. Irani S, Arai A, Ayub K, et al. Papillectomy for ampullary neoplasm: results of a single referral center over a 10-year period. Gastrointest Endosc 2009;70: 923–32.
31. Yamao T, Isomoto H, Kohno S, et al. Endoscopic snare papillectomy with biliary and pancreatic stent placement for tumors of the major duodenal papilla. Surg Endosc 2010;24:119–24.
32. Ito K, Fujita N, Noda Y. Endoscopic diagnosis and treatment of ampullary neoplasm (with video). Dig Endosc 2011;23:113–7.
33. Artifon EL, Couto D Jr, Sakai P, et al. Prospective evaluation of EUS versus CT scan for staging of ampullary cancer. Gastrointest Endosc 2009;70:290–6.

34. Sauvanet A, Chapuis O, Hammel P, et al. Are endoscopic procedures able to predict the benignity of ampullary tumors? Am J Surg 1997;174:355–8.
35. Chen CH, Yang CC, Yeh YH, et al. Reappraisal of endosonography of ampullary tumors: correlation with transabdominal sonography, CT, and MRI. J Clin Ultrasound 2009;37:18–25.
36. Rosch T, Braig C, Gain T, et al. Staging of pancreatic and ampullary carcinoma by endoscopic ultrasonography. Comparison with conventional sonography, computed tomography, and angiography. Gastroenterology 1992;102:188–99.
37. Cannon ME, Carpenter SL, Elta GH, et al. EUS compared with CT, magnetic resonance imaging, and angiography and the influence of biliary stenting on staging accuracy of ampullary neoplasms. Gastrointest Endosc 1999;50:27–33.
38. Manta R, Conigliaro R, Castellani D, et al. Linear endoscopic ultrasonography vs magnetic resonance imaging in ampullary tumors. World J Gastroenterol 2010;16:5592–7.
39. Tio TL, Sie LH, Kallimanis G, et al. Staging of ampullary and pancreatic carcinoma: comparison between endosonography and surgery. Gastrointest Endosc 1996;44:706–13.
40. Itoh A, Goto H, Naitoh Y, et al. Intraductal ultrasonography in diagnosing tumor extension of cancer of the papilla of Vater. Gastrointest Endosc 1997;45:251–60.
41. Menzel J, Hoepffner N, Sulkowski U, et al. Polypoid tumors of the major duodenal papilla: preoperative staging with intraductal US, EUS, and CT–a prospective, histopathologically controlled study. Gastrointest Endosc 1999;49:349–57.
42. Ito K, Fujita N, Noda Y, et al. Preoperative evaluation of ampullary neoplasm with EUS and transpapillary intraductal US: a prospective and histopathologically controlled study. Gastrointest Endosc 2007;66:740–7.
43. Sivak MV. Clinical and endoscopic aspects of tumors of the ampulla of Vater. Endoscopy 1988;20(Suppl 1):211–7.
44. Ito K, Fujita N, Noda Y, et al. Case of early ampullary cancer treated by endoscopic papillectomy. Dig Endosc 2004;16:157–61.
45. Standards of Practice ASGE Committee, Adler DG, Qureshi W, et al. The role of endoscopy in ampullary and duodenal adenomas. Gastrointest Endosc 2006;64:849–54.
46. Han J, Kim MH. Endoscopic papillectomy for adenomas of the major duodenal papilla. Gastrointest Endosc 2006;63:292–301.
47. Chini P, Draganov P. Diagnosis and management of ampullary adenoma: the expanding role of endoscopy. World J Gastrointest Endosc 2011;3:241–7.
48. Aiura K, Imaeda H, Kitajima M, et al. Balloon-catheter-assisted endoscopic snare papillectomy for benign tumors of the major duodenal papilla. Gastrointest Endosc 2003;57:743–7.
49. Ito K, Fujita N, Noda Y, et al. Impact of technical modification of endoscopic papillectomy for ampullary neoplasm on the occurrence of complications. Dig Endosc 2012;24:30–5.
50. Saurin JC, Chavaillon A, Napoleon B, et al. Long-term follow-up of patients with endoscopic treatment of sporadic adenomas of the papilla of Vater. Endoscopy 2003;35:402–6.
51. Lee SK, Kim MH, Seo DW, et al. Endoscopic sphincterotomy and pancreatic duct placement before endoscopic papillectomy: are they necessary and safe procedure? Gastrointest Endosc 2002;55:302–4.
52. Kennan J, Mallery S, Freeman ML. EUS rendezvous for pancreatic stent placement during endoscopic snare ampullectomy. Gastrointest Endosc 2007;66:850–3.

53. Choi JJ, Kim MH, Kim GD, et al. Papillary stenosis and cholangitis caused by endoscopic mucosal resection of ampullary adenoma. Korean J Gastrointest Endosc 2003;27:249–53.
54. Baillie J. Endoscopic ampullectomy: does pancreatic stent placement make it safer? Gastrointest Endosc 2005;62:371–3.
55. Moon J, Cha S, Cho Y, et al. Wire-guided endoscopic snare papillectomy for tumors of the major duodenal papilla. Gastrointest Endosc 2005;61:461–6.
56. Kim JH, Moon JH, Choi HJ, et al. Endoscopic snare papillectomy by using a balloon catheter for an unexposed empullary adenoma with intraductal extension. Gastrointest Endosc 2009;69:1404–6.
57. Fukushima H, Yamamato H, Nakano H, et al. Complete en bloc resection of a large scale ampullary adenoma with a focal adenocarcinoma by using endoscopic submucosal dissection. Gastrointest Endosc 2009;70:592–5.

Small Bowel Polyps, Arteriovenous Malformations, Strictures, and Miscellaneous Lesions

Rahul Pannala, MD[a], Andrew S. Ross, MD[b],*

KEYWORDS

- Endoscopy • Small intestine • Peutz-Jeghers syndrome
- Arteriovenous malformations • Enteral stents

KEY POINTS

- In the era of intraoperative enteroscopy, the endoscopist has access to a plethora of new endoscopes and devices, which have significantly altered the therapeutic modalities that can be applied deep within the small intestine.
- The need for intraoperative enteroscopy or surgical resection of small bowel has been significantly decreased (and in some cases, eliminated) by the application of these technologies in clinical practice.
- This field remains in evolution and the future will undoubtedly include the design of new instruments that may help overcome many of the technical limitations associated with performing therapeutic maneuvers deep within the small intestine.

INTRODUCTION

Advances in endoscopic techniques and the availability of newer endoscopes and accessories have allowed for exciting new applications of therapeutic endoscopy within the small intestine. Many procedures that were previously the purview of surgery are now performed endoscopically. This article provides an overview of the current endoscopic management of small bowel polyps, arteriovenous malformations (AVMs), strictures, and miscellaneous lesions identified within the small intestine.

Disclosures: None.
[a] Division of Gastroenterology and Hepatology, Mayo Clinic, 13400 East Shea Boulevard, Scottsdale, AZ 85259, USA; [b] Digestive Disease Institute, Virginia Mason Medical Center, 1100 9th Avenue, Seattle, WA 98101, USA
* Corresponding author.
E-mail address: Andrew.ross@vmmc.org

GENERAL PRINCIPLES OF ENDOLUMENAL THERAPY IN THE SMALL BOWEL

The primary challenge for endoscopic interventions in the small bowel is access to the lesions, particularly past the proximal jejunum. Endoscopic interventions in the proximal duodenum are usually performed with regular or therapeutic upper endoscopes or duodenoscopes. Previously, deeper access into the small bowel was achieved with the use of a pediatric colonoscope or a push enteroscope, which could be advanced to the proximal jejunum. More distal lesions would require intraoperative enteroscopy with significant associated morbidity.

In the past decade, the introduction of single-balloon (SBE) (Olympus Corporation, Tokyo, Japan) and double-balloon enteroscopes (DBE) (Fujinon Inc, Saitama, Japan) and rotational enteroscopy (RE) (Spirus Medical Inc, Stoughton, MA, USA) has substantially improved deep access into the small bowel so that most lesions are accessible endoscopically. These devices allow for access to the small bowel either per os or per rectum. Therefore, having an estimate of the approximate location of the lesion of interest before embarking on endoscopy is critical. Today, most deep enteroscopy is directed by capsule endoscopy,[1] although CT or MRI can also be used.

Although location and the ability to reach the lesion are critical, other factors may define whether a lesion in the small bowel can be approached endoscopically. Position and endoscope control are critical to performing therapeutic endoscopy. Optimizing these 2 factors deep within the small intestine can occasionally present a significant challenge. Another key aspect of therapeutic intervention in the small bowel is availability and selection of endoscopic accessories. Currently, most of the accessories required for endolumenal therapy of polyps, vascular lesions, and strictures (snares, thermal devices, dilation balloons, and clips) are either long enough (>230 cm) or are available in the enteroscopy length. However, the length of the enteroscope (2 m) and the limited diameter (2.8 mm) of the accessory channel combined with significant looping can make the use of these accessories difficult. Loop reduction through shortening the endoscope before attempting therapy greatly improves the ability to pass accessories through the scope channel and perform successful interventions.

SMALL BOWEL POLYPS

Sporadic small bowel polyps are rare and usually found incidentally on endoscopy. The prevalence of sporadic duodenal polyps is estimated to be 4.6% of all patients undergoing diagnostic endoscopy.[2] These polyps are usually asymptomatic but can occasionally present with bleeding or abdominal pain.[3] Ampullary adenomas are usually also discovered incidentally but can present with biliary colic or obstructive jaundice, or can be suspected on cross-sectional imaging if biliary or pancreatic ductal dilation up to the level of the ampulla is noted. Otherwise, small bowel polyps are usually encountered in the setting of polyposis syndromes, such as Peutz-Jeghers syndrome (PJS) or familial adenomatous polyposis syndrome (FAP).

PJS

PJS is an autosomal dominant genetic disorder whose gene locus has been mapped to chromosome 19p13.3, which is a serine threonine kinase gene known as LKB1 or STK11.[4] The syndrome manifests as hamartomatous polyps in the gastrointestinal tract, mucocutaneous pigmentation, and an increased risk of gastrointestinal and other cancers.[5] Hamartomas in PJS are primarily located within the small bowel, and clinical diagnosis of PJS is usually related to a manifestation of bowel hamartomas, such as small bowel obstruction from intussusception, abdominal pain, rectal bleeding, and polyp extrusion.[6] In a study involving 222 patients with PJS, 49% had gastric polyps, 64% had small bowel polyps, 53% had colon polyps, and 32% had rectal polyps.[7] In one series, the lifetime intussusception risk was approximately 70%, with a 50% intussusception risk by the age of 20 years[6]; 95% of the intussusceptions occurred in the small bowel, and among small bowel intussusception events, 53% occurred in the jejunum and 47% were within the ileum. The hamartomas associated with small bowel intussusception were also noted to be larger than 15 mm, with a median size of 35 mm.

Patients with PJS are also at a substantial risk for gastrointestinal and other malignancies. The risk of gastrointestinal cancer is estimated to be between 38% and 66%, with 39% occurring in the colon and rectum, 29% in the stomach, 13% in the small bowel, and 11% to 36% in the pancreas.[8]

The objectives of screening and surveillance for polyps in PJS include the prevention of obstruction, intussusception, and cancer.[5] Upper endoscopy and colonoscopy are used to evaluate the upper and lower gastrointestinal tract, but evaluation of the small bowel can be challenging. Video capsule endoscopy and MR enterography are the preferred modalities for screening and surveillance of small bowel polyps, although small bowel series and CT enterography are often used. The goals of endoscopic therapy are to resect polyps that are larger than 15 mm, because these pose the highest risk for intussusception.[6]

Endoscopic polypectomy for small bowel PJS polyps can be performed using DBE, SBE, or RE (**Fig. 1**). In a prospective series of 13 patients with PJS, Gao and colleagues[9] described a total of 82 polyps 1 cm or larger; polyps were predominantly

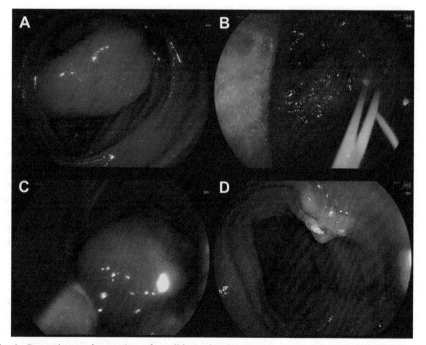

Fig. 1. Detection and resection of small bowel polyp in PJS at DBE. (*A*) Typical appearance of PJS polyps, which predispose to intussusception. (*B*) Placement of endoloop at base of polyp before resection. (*C*) Snare cautery. (*D*) Postpolypectomy site. (*Courtesy of* Dr. Shabana F. Pasha, Scottsdale, Arizona.)

noted in the proximal jejunum (94%). Most patients (77%) underwent a previous partial bowel resection for small bowel polyps. In this group, a total of 29 DBE procedures were performed, and 79 of 82 polyps (96%) were resected without any major complications. After endoscopic resection and a follow-up of 356 person-months, no small bowel–related complications were seen and none of the patients required surgery. Similar results were also noted in another series of 15 patients with PJS from Japan.[10] This series also reported that the average size of the polyps decreased with successive endoscopies.

A hybrid approach using a laparoscopy-assisted DBE with complete enteroscopy and polypectomy of all lesions greater than 0.5 cm has also been described.[11] Many patients with PJS have had previous bowel resections, and angulation from adhesions may make enteroscopy challenging. In these instances, a combined endoscopic and surgical approach may be suitable for complete examination of the small bowel. In centers in which balloon-assisted enteroscopy is not available, intraoperative endoscopy for clearance of small bowel polyps is a reasonable approach. Surgical resection remains the mainstay for patients with PJS who present with acute obstruction, intussusception, and large polyps not amenable to endoscopic resection.[5]

Current surveillance guidelines for PJS recommend baseline small bowel video capsule endoscopy at the age of 8 years, or earlier if the patient is symptomatic.[5] If polyps are identified on baseline video capsule endoscopy, this procedure should be repeated every 3 years. If few or no polyps are found on initial video capsule endoscopy, small bowel screening should resume at 3-year intervals beginning at 18 years of age, or sooner if symptoms develop. MR and CT enterography and conventional small bowel contrast radiography using barium have been proposed as alternatives when video capsule endoscopy is not available or is contraindicated.

In addition to PJS, small bowel polyps are also occasionally encountered in other hamartomatous polyposis syndromes, such as juvenile polyposis syndrome and PTEN hamartoma tumor syndrome, which includes Cowden, Bannayan-Zonana, and Proteus syndromes.[12]

FAP

The duodenum is the most common site for adenomas in FAP after the colon.[12,13] Nearly 65% of FAP patients will have a duodenal adenoma at their first endoscopy (median age, 35 years), and over time virtually all patients develop a duodenal adenoma, with more than a half having an advanced adenoma. Consequently, these patients have a markedly higher risk of duodenal and periampullary adenocarcinoma, and this is the leading cause of death in these patients.[14] Therefore, patients with FAP are recommended to have surveillance endoscopies, including a side-viewing examination of the ampulla every 1 to 2 years. Endoscopic treatment of duodenal and ampullary adenomas is a crucial aspect of the care of these patients. The management of ampullary adenomas is discussed in detail elsewhere in this issue by El Hajj and Coté.

Nonampullary Duodenal Polyps

Nonampullary duodenal polyps are usually detected incidentally at upper endoscopy, and their prevalence ranges from 1 to 3 per 1000.[3] These polyps are also seen in the setting of polyposis syndromes, such as PJS and FAP. Most of these polyps can resected endoscopically using a technique of submucosal injection followed by snare resection.[15] Endoloop placement may be helpful for thick pedunculated polyps. Argon plasma coagulation is commonly used to ablate the borders of the polypectomy or remaining polypoid tissue. Surgery is reserved for lesions that are not amenable to endoscopic resection or in the presence of evidence of malignancy with submucosal invasion.[16]

In a series of 62 patients treated for nonampullary duodenal polyps over the course of 10 years from 1990 through 2000, Perez and colleagues[17] reported that most patients (47/62, 76%) were treated endoscopically and 15 patients underwent surgery. Major morbidity was seen in 1 of 47 patients treated endoscopically compared with 5 of 15 patients treated surgically (P = .002). Surgically treated patients expectedly had a higher median polyp diameter compared with those treated endoscopically (35 vs 8 mm, respectively; $P<.01$). In another series of 59 patients,[18] the mean polyp size was 17.2 ± 1.6 mm, and complete endoscopic resection was achieved in 98% of these polyps. Polyps greater than 2 cm were more likely to recur after endoscopic resection. Another study compared endoscopic resection of giant hemicircumferential lateral-spreading tumors (mean size, 4 cm; range, 3–8 cm) with smaller duodenal adenomas (<3 cm) and reported that endoscopic resection was safe and effective even in these challenging lesions.[19] The incidence of bleeding complications was higher in the larger tumors than in the smaller tumors (26% vs 3%; P = .01).

Collectively, these studies indicate that endoscopic resection is safe and effective for most duodenal adenomas. However, it is associated with a higher rate of complications, particularly bleeding (both early and delayed), than is typically observed with polypectomy at other sites in the gastrointestinal tract. Recurrence is common, and therefore endoscopic surveillance is routinely performed.

AVMS

Bleeding, particularly obscure gastrointestinal bleeding, is one of the most common indications for enteroscopy.[20] According to some estimates, obscure gastrointestinal bleeding, which by definition is bleeding that occurs between the ligament of Treitz and the ileocecal valve, AVMs (angioectasia) are the most likely sources of bleeding from the small intestine, especially in older patients.[21] Other sources of bleeding from the small bowel are Dieulafoy lesions (see later discussion), tumors, varices, ulcers, and Meckel diverticulum. Most commonly, enteroscopy is performed after a negative upper endoscopy and colonoscopy. Capsule endoscopy or, less commonly, CT or MR enterography are usually performed before enteroscopy to identify the location and extent of the bleeding lesions, and to allow for the selection of the appropriate route of initial endoscope access (**Fig. 2**).[1] Although capsule-directed deep enteroscopy for obscure gastrointestinal bleeding has become the accepted norm in most patients when this technology is available, Monkemuller and colleagues[22] showed the feasibility of urgent DBE in the setting of overt obscure gastrointestinal bleeding and were able to identify and treat bleeding lesions in 9 of 10 patients (90%).

AVMs are usually treated by argon plasma coagulation, and enteroscopy-length probes for argon plasma coagulation are available and effective.[15,23] Gerson and colleagues[24] reported long-term outcomes of 40 patients with AVMs treated with argon plasma coagulation at DBE for overt or obscure gastrointestinal bleeding. At 1 year, 17 (43%) patients had no recurrence of bleeding or the need for iron or transfusions, 11 (28%) had recurrence of overt bleeding, and 12 (30%) reported the need for iron or transfusion therapy. In this study, 30-month follow-up data on 29 patients with AVMs showed that 16 (55%) patients had no further bleeding and 13 (45%) reported overt bleeding or the need for iron or transfusions despite treatment. Samaha and colleagues[25] reported similar results in a cohort of 133 patients with small bowel

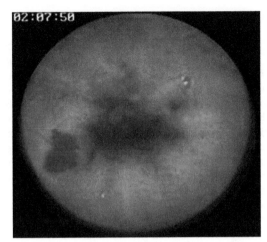
02:07:50

Fig. 2. Angioectasia detected at capsule endoscopy, which is routinely used before entero-scopy to localize and assess the extent of the bleeding lesions.

capsular lesions treated with DBE; after a median of 22.6 months, the rebleeding rate was 46%. Other techniques for treatment of AVMs include endoscopic clip placement and thermal therapy with bipolar or heater probes.

Other factors, including the use of antiplatelet agents and anticoagulation, may increase the risk of bleeding from small bowel AVMs. Based on available data, a significant number of patients will experience rebleeding even after treatment of AVMs at enteroscopy, and therefore a careful review of other factors that may influence rebleeding, such as medications, should be undertaken at patient consultation. Finally, patients with obscure gastrointestinal bleeding secondary to small bowel AVMs should be counseled regarding the significant rate of rebleeding so as to set appropriate expectations.

SMALL BOWEL STRICTURES

Strictures of the small intestine are typically seen in the setting of small bowel Crohn disease or with use of nonsteroidal anti-inflammatory drugs (NSAIDs) (**Fig. 3**).[26,27] Other causes include radiation enteritis, previous small bowel surgeries, and ischemia. These patients usually present with symptoms of partial small bowel obstruction. Strictures or webs are identified on CT or MR enterography or video capsule endos-copy, but these can be subtle and missed on imaging. Unsuspected strictures can lead to capsule retention with subsequent need for endoscopic or surgical removal.[28] As with small bowel polyps, the emergence of therapeutic deep enteroscopy has decreased the need for surgery in the management of these strictures.

Balloon Strictureplasty

Successful balloon dilation of NSAID strictures and strictures from Crohn disease has been reported. Ohmiya and colleagues[27] reported outcomes of 47 balloon dilations performed through DBE in 22 patients with various diseases and noted that 96% were successful. In this study, 16 patients had Crohn disease and among them, 11 (69%) remained asymptomatic after dilation. Through the scope, balloon dilators to a maximum of 20 mm were used. Perforation was reported in only one patient.

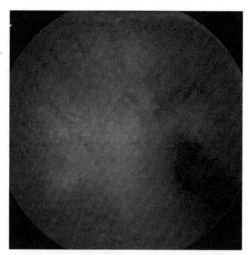

Fig. 3. Capsule endoscopic view of a small bowel stricture from nonsteroidal-related diaphragm disease. Unsuspected diaphragm disease can lead to capsule retention and require enteroscopic or surgical removal.

Several other smaller studies have also reported favorable outcomes with balloon strictureplasty.[29,30]

In strictures caused by Crohn disease, only fibrostenotic strictures are amenable to dilation, and the presence of active inflammation is usually considered a contraindication to dilation.[27] Patients with Crohn disease typically have had multiple previous abdominal surgeries, which result in adhesions. Intestinal angulation and fixation from adhesions can limit the reach of the enteroscope and increase the risk of perforation. Some of these patients may also have multiple sites of stricturing, which can make therapy challenging. Nevertheless, a meta-analysis including 347 patients with Crohn disease undergoing balloon strictureplasty reported technical success in 86% of patients, with 58% of patients reporting long-term efficacy after a median follow-up of 33 months.[31] The rate of major complications (ie, perforation) was 2%.

Several technical aspects deserve mention in balloon dilation of small bowel strictures. A colonic-length (240 cm) balloon dilator should be used with the enteroscopes.[15] The limited diameter of the DBE or SBE working channel makes the balloon dilator difficult to pass, especially in the setting of looping. As with the passage of other accessories, reduction maneuvers are helpful. Lubricating the channel with silicone can also be attempted. Care should also be taken to avoid bending the balloon catheter during passage through the enteroscope, because this makes further passage of the instrument difficult.

As with Crohn disease, endoscopic balloon dilation of NSAID-related diaphragm disease has also been successful.[28] Capsule retention can be a challenging problem in patients with diaphragm disease; DBE can also be helpful in this regard to retrieve the capsule and avoid surgery.

ENTERAL STENTS

Self-expanding metal stents (SEMS) are effective for palliation of malignant gastric outlet and duodenal obstruction.[32] Their use farther distally in the small bowel has been limited by both the difficulty with access beyond the distal duodenum and the flexibility and length of stent delivery systems. SEMS placement in the distal duodenum and proximal jejunum with the DBE scope and Spirus overtube has been reported.[33,34] However, the working channel of the DBE is too small to accommodate currently available through-the-scope enteral stents.[33] In these reports, reduction of the gastric and early small bowel looping enabled the passage of the endoscope to the point of the stenosis at which the overtube balloon was inflated to hold position, the endoscope was removed, and the stent deployed through the overtube under fluoroscopic guidance. If the endoscope can be passed beyond the stricture, it is helpful to place and endoclip to mark the distal end of the stricture for more precise stent placement (**Fig. 4**). However, these procedures remain challenging and a distinct need exists for the development of dedicated stent delivery systems designed for the enteroscope.

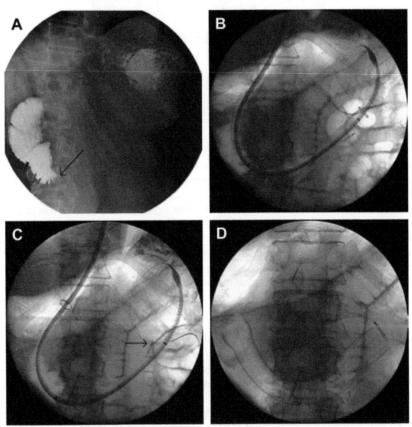

Fig. 4. Enteral stent placement using double-balloon enteroscopy. (*A*) Small bowel series showing distal duodenal obstruction (*arrow*). (*B*) Fluoroscopy showing passage of the stent delivery system through the overtube of the DBE scope. Image also shows placement of an endoclip to mark the distal aspect of the stricture (*arrow*). (*C*) Stent delivery system is maintained in position as the overtube is removed from the patient. (*D*) Fluoroscopic image showing expanded stent deployed across the stricture. (*Modified from* Ross A, Semrad C, Waxman I, et al. Enteral stent placement by double balloon enteroscopy for palliation of malignant small bowel obstruction. Gastrointest Endosc 2006;64(5):835-7 with permission.)

MISCELLANEOUS LESIONS
Dieulafoy Lesions

Dieulafoy lesions consist of superficial ulceration with an exposed aberrant submucosal artery and can account for severe gastrointestinal bleeding. These lesions accounted for 3.5% of patients who had an SBE or DBE for mid-gastrointestinal bleeding, and were most commonly noted in the proximal jejunum.[35] Various endoscopic hemostatic techniques can be used, but endoclips may be preferable to argon plasma coagulation in the setting of a pulsatile vascular lesion such as a Dieulafoy lesion.[23]

Small Bowel Tumors

Small bowel tumors are rare, accounting for only 2% of primary gastrointestinal malignancies.[36] Although video capsule endoscopy and radiologic enterography techniques have substantially improved the diagnosis and localization of these tumors, diagnosis remains a challenge.[37] Deep enteroscopy can be extremely helpful in localizing these tumors, performing endoscopic biopsies to establish diagnosis, tattooing the site for operative localization, and, in selected cases, performing endoscopic resection.

SUMMARY

In the era of intraoperative enteroscopy, the modern endoscopist has access to a plethora of new endoscopes and devices, which have significantly altered the therapeutic modalities that can be applied deep within the small intestine. The need for intraoperative enteroscopy or surgical resection of the small bowel has been significantly decreased (and in some cases, eliminated) through the application of these technologies in clinical practice. Clearly, this remains a field in evolution, and the future will undoubtedly include the design of new instruments that may help overcome many of the technical limitations associated with performing therapeutic maneuvers deep within the small intestine.

REFERENCES

1. Gay G, Delvaux M. Small-bowel endoscopy. Endoscopy 2006;38(1):22–6.
2. Jepsen JM, Persson M, Jakobsen NO, et al. Prospective study of prevalence and endoscopic and histopathologic characteristics of duodenal polyps in patients submitted to upper endoscopy. Scand J Gastroenterol 1994;29(6):483–7.
3. Culver EL, McIntyre AS. Sporadic duodenal polyps: classification, investigation, and management. Endoscopy 2011;43(2):144–55.
4. Hemminki A, Tomlinson I, Markie D, et al. Localization of a susceptibility locus for Peutz-Jeghers syndrome to 19p using comparative genomic hybridization and targeted linkage analysis. Nat Genet 1997;15(1):87–90.
5. Beggs AD, Latchford AR, Vasen HF, et al. Peutz-Jeghers syndrome: a systematic review and recommendations for management. Gut 2010;59(7):975–86.
6. van Lier MG, Mathus-Vliegen EM, Wagner A, et al. High cumulative risk of intussusception in patients with Peutz-Jeghers syndrome: time to update surveillance guidelines? Am J Gastroenterol 2011;106(5):940–5.
7. Utsunomiya J, Gocho H, Miyanaga T, et al. Peutz-Jeghers syndrome: its natural course and management. Johns Hopkins Med J 1975;136(2):71–82.
8. Boardman LA, Thibodeau SN, Schaid DJ, et al. Increased risk for cancer in patients with the Peutz-Jeghers syndrome. Ann Intern Med 1998;128(11):896–9.

9. Gao H, van Lier MG, Poley JW, et al. Endoscopic therapy of small-bowel polyps by double-balloon enteroscopy in patients with Peutz-Jeghers syndrome. Gastrointest Endosc 2010;71(4):768–73.

10. Sakamoto H, Yamamoto H, Hayashi Y, et al. Nonsurgical management of small-bowel polyps in Peutz-Jeghers syndrome with extensive polypectomy by using double-balloon endoscopy. Gastrointest Endosc 2011;74(2):328–33.

11. Ross AS, Dye C, Prachand VN. Laparoscopic-assisted double-balloon enteroscopy for small-bowel polyp surveillance and treatment in patients with Peutz-Jeghers syndrome. Gastrointest Endosc 2006;64(6):984–8.

12. Arber N, Moshkowitz M. Small bowel polyposis syndromes. Curr Gastroenterol Rep 2011;13(5):435–41.

13. Bulow S, Bjork J, Christensen IJ, et al. Duodenal adenomatosis in familial adenomatous polyposis. Gut 2004;53(3):381–6.

14. Laurent S, Franchimont D, Coppens JP, et al. Familial adenomatous polyposis: clinical presentation, detection and surveillance. Acta Gastroenterol Belg 2011;74(3):415–20.

15. Kaffes AJ. Advances in modern enteroscopy therapeutics. Best Pract Res Clin Gastroenterol 2012;26(3):235–46.

16. van Heumen BW, Nieuwenhuis MH, van Goor H, et al. Surgical management for advanced duodenal adenomatosis and duodenal cancer in Dutch patients with familial adenomatous polyposis: a nationwide retrospective cohort study. Surgery 2012;151(5):681–90.

17. Perez A, Saltzman JR, Carr-Locke DL, et al. Benign nonampullary duodenal neoplasms. J Gastrointest Surg 2003;7(4):536–41.

18. Abbass R, Rigaux J, Al-Kawas FH. Nonampullary duodenal polyps: characteristics and endoscopic management. Gastrointest Endosc 2010;71(4):754–9.

19. Fanning SB, Bourke MJ, Williams SJ, et al. Giant laterally spreading tumors of the duodenum: endoscopic resection outcomes, limitations, and caveats. Gastrointest Endosc 2012;75(4):805–12.

20. Jeon SR, Kim JO, Kim HG, et al. Changes over time in indications, diagnostic yield, and clinical effects of double-balloon enteroscopy. Clin Gastroenterol Hepatol 2012;10(10):1152–6.

21. Yano T, Yamamoto H. Vascular, polypoid, and other lesions of the small bowel. Best Pract Res Clin Gastroenterol 2009;23(1):61–74.

22. Monkemuller K, Neumann H, Meyer F, et al. A retrospective analysis of emergency double-balloon enteroscopy for small-bowel bleeding. Endoscopy 2009; 41(8):715–7.

23. Raju GS, Gerson L, Das A, et al. American Gastroenterological Association (AGA) Institute technical review on obscure gastrointestinal bleeding. Gastroenterology 2007;133(5):1697–717.

24. Gerson LB, Batenic MA, Newsom SL, et al. Long-term outcomes after double-balloon enteroscopy for obscure gastrointestinal bleeding. Clin Gastroenterol Hepatol 2009;7(6):664–9.

25. Samaha E, Rahmi G, Landi B, et al. Long-term outcome of patients treated with double balloon enteroscopy for small bowel vascular lesions. Am J Gastroenterol 2012;107(2):240–6.

26. May A, Nachbar L, Pohl J, et al. Endoscopic interventions in the small bowel using double balloon enteroscopy: feasibility and limitations. Am J Gastroenterol 2007;102(3):527–35.

27. Ohmiya N, Arakawa D, Nakamura M, et al. Small-bowel obstruction: diagnostic comparison between double-balloon endoscopy and fluoroscopic enteroclysis, and the outcome of enteroscopic treatment. Gastrointest Endosc 2009;69(1):84–93.

28. Mehdizadeh S, Lo SK. Treatment of small-bowel diaphragm disease by using double-balloon enteroscopy. Gastrointest Endosc 2006;64(6):1014–7.
29. Hirai F, Beppu T, Sou S, et al. Endoscopic balloon dilatation using double-balloon endoscopy is a useful and safe treatment for small intestinal strictures in Crohn's disease. Dig Endosc 2010;22(3):200–4.
30. Despott EJ, Gupta A, Burling D, et al. Effective dilation of small-bowel strictures by double-balloon enteroscopy in patients with symptomatic Crohn's disease (with video). Gastrointest Endosc 2009;70(5):1030–6.
31. Hassan C, Zullo A, De Francesco V, et al. Systematic review: endoscopic dilatation in Crohn's disease. Aliment Pharmacol Ther 2007;26(11–12):1457–64.
32. Varadarajulu S, Banerjee S, Barth B, et al. Enteral stents. Gastrointest Endosc 2011;74(3):455–64.
33. Ross AS, Semrad C, Waxman I, et al. Enteral stent placement by double balloon enteroscopy for palliation of malignant small bowel obstruction. Gastrointest Endosc 2006;64(5):835–7.
34. Lennon AM, Chandrasekhara V, Shin EJ, et al. Spiral-enteroscopy-assisted enteral stent placement for palliation of malignant small-bowel obstruction (with video). Gastrointest Endosc 2010;71(2):422–5.
35. Dulic-Lakovic E, Dulic M, Hubner D, et al. Bleeding Dieulafoy lesions of the small bowel: a systematic study on the epidemiology and efficacy of enteroscopic treatment. Gastrointest Endosc 2011;74(3):573–80.
36. Paski SC, Semrad CE. Small bowel tumors. Gastrointest Endosc Clin N Am 2009; 19(3):461–79.
37. Ross A, Mehdizadeh S, Tokar J, et al. Double balloon enteroscopy detects small bowel mass lesions missed by capsule endoscopy. Dig Dis Sci 2008;53(8): 2140–3.

Endoscopic Therapy for Postoperative Leaks and Fistulae

Nitin Kumar, MD[a], Christopher C. Thompson, MD, MSc[b],*

KEYWORDS

- Endoscopy • Endoscopic • Bariatric • Fistula • Leak • Surgery • Postoperative
- Stent

KEY POINTS

- Endoscopic techniques for the treatment of postoperative fistulae and leaks are rapidly developing.
- Conventional surgical therapy for postsurgical leaks and fistulae is associated with significant morbidity and mortality.
- Novel endoscopic therapies, such as endoscopic suturing, novel stent types, and vacuum-assisted sponge closure, have demonstrated safety and are building evidence for efficacy.
- We examine endoscopic therapy for leaks and fistulae after esophageal, gastric, bariatric, colonic, and pancreaticobiliary surgery.

INTRODUCTION

Endoscopic techniques for the diagnosis and therapy for gastrointestinal disease are rapidly developing. Fistulae are abnormal communications originating in a visceral structure. Postoperative leaks are 1 type of fistula, defined as discontinuity of tissue apposition in the immediate postoperative period. Conventional surgical therapy for postsurgical leaks and fistulae is associated with significant morbidity and mortality, and new endoscopic options offer significant benefits. This article examines endoscopic therapy for leaks and fistulae after esophageal, gastric, bariatric, colonic, and pancreaticobiliary surgery.

Disclosures: Nitin Kumar: None. Christopher C. Thompson: Boston Scientific – Consultant (Consulting fees). USGI Medical – Consultant (Consulting Fees)/Advisory Board Member (Travel and attendance fees). Valentx – Consultant (Consulting Fees). Olympus – Lab Support (Lab supplies/equipment), Consultant. Vysera – Consultant, Lab support. Beacon Endoscopic – Consultant/Stock. Apollo Endosurgery – Consultant. Barosense - Consultant.
[a] Division of Gastroenterology, Brigham and Women's Hospital, 75 Francis Street, Boston, MA 02115, USA; [b] Division of Gastroenterology, Brigham and Women's Hospital, 75 Francis Street, ASB II, Boston, MA 02115, USA
* Corresponding author.
E-mail address: christopher_thompson@hms.harvard.edu

ESOPHAGEAL LEAKS AND FISTULAE
Scope of the Problem

Postoperative esophageal leaks and fistulae can develop after esophagectomy or gastrectomy. The intrathoracic leak rate after esophageal resection has been reported at 7.9%, resulting in a 3-month mortality rate of 18.2% (OR 3.0).[1] If treatment is delayed beyond the first 24 hours, a mortality rate has been reported at up to 50%.[2] Esophageal leakage after gastrectomy occurs in 4% to 27%, and a mortality rate of 65% has been reported.[3,4]

Past Management Options

Surgical therapy for postoperative leak historically consisted of surgical drainage and repair, nothing by mouth, parenteral nutrition, and antibiotics. The result was a mortality rate of up to 60%.[5] Fever, systemic inflammatory response syndrome, and abnormal C-reactive protein, white blood cell count, and albumin are indicators of postoperative esophageal leak.[6,7]

Current Status

Early diagnosis is important to prevent fulminant infection. Endoscopy is useful in diagnosis because the defect, integrity of surrounding tissue, and infection in the adjacent tissue can be assessed; these factors are important in choosing treatment modality. Fibrin glue or endoscopic clip placement can be considered for small defects, although patients with dehiscence of 30% to 70% of the esophageal circumference likely warrant stent placement. Larger defects are not amenable to endoscopic therapy.

Esophageal stent placement for postoperative fistula and leak has become well-established. Both covered self-expanding metal stents (SEMS) and self-expanding plastic stents (SEPS) have been studied. Stent placement excludes the defect to allow healing, prevents stricture formation, and may allow oral feeding. However, stent placement can be complicated by inadequate defect closure, stent migration, and difficult removal caused by tissue ingrowth or stricture. Leaks at an anastomosis where the esophagus is contiguous with small intestine or colon are challenging candidates for stent placement because of the risk of necrosis and migration, respectively. Freeman and colleagues[8] recently reported that factors associated with failure of leak resolution after stent placement included leak of the proximal cervical esophagus, stent traversing the gastroesophageal junction, esophageal injury greater than 6 cm, and anastomotic leak associated with a more distal conduit leak.

New Endolumenal Options

Novel stents have been used to close postoperative esophageal leaks and fistulae. A covered biodegradable stent, which does not need to be removed after therapy completion or migration, has demonstrated leak closure in 4 of 5 patients.[9] A mushroom-shaped metallic stent has been used successfully for durable treatment of gastroesophageal anastomotic fistula in 8 of 8 patients, with successful removal in within 48 days.[10]

Endoscopic clips can be used to close fistulae and leaks. Clips are deployed perpendicular to the long axis of the defect to approximate the edges of the defect. Multiple clips can be placed beginning at either edge of a defect and meeting at the center. Mechanical scraping or thermal ablation of the defect edges before clip placement results in a more durable seal.[11] Luminal distention should be avoided before and after clip placement. The Over the Scope Clip (OTSC; Ovesco Endoscopy

AG, Tübingen, Germany) is a nitinol clip deployed from a cap at the endoscope tip after tissue is suctioned into the cap.[12] The OTSC can perform full-thickness apposition, unlike through-the-scope clips.[13] Case series have shown success rates of 72% to 91% for gastrointestinal tract fistula closure.[12,14,15] Success has been reported for initial closure of postoperative esophagojejunal anastomotic leaks and fistulae.[12,16]

Sealants have been used to treat postoperative esophageal leaks. N-butyl-2-cyano-acrylate (Histoacryl; B. Braun Dexon GmbH, Spangenberg, Germany) has been successfully used to repair an esophagojejunal anastomotic leak after 3 weeks of conservative therapy failed.[17] Fibrin glue, which has a long history of surgical use, has been used to close an esophageal fistula via submucosal injection into the lateral walls of the fistula rather than injection into the fistula.[18] The glue is injected into the submucosa until the lumen is occluded, ensuring that the fibrin plug does not become dislodged. No abrasion or deepithelialization of the fistula tract is required. Vicryl mesh (Ethicon, Hamburg, German) has been combined with use of fibrin sealant for closure of larger postoperative leaks or fistulae.[19] After the mesh is placed over the defect, it is covered with 2 to 3 mL fibrin (Tissucol Duo, Baxter, Germany), and then fibrin is injected into the submucosa at the edges of the defect. The defect eventually epithelializes. Thirteen of 15 patients had long-term success with this technique. Surgisis Soft Tissue Graft (Cook, West Lafayette, IN), an acellular bioactive prosthetic matrix, has been used successfully in conjunction with the OTSC and SEMS (**Fig. 1**).[20]

Vacuum-assisted sponge closure (VAC) therapy has been investigated for closure of esophageal defects. Because negative intrathoracic pressure can draw fluid through even small defects with each inspiration, intrathoracic collections and infection can develop. VAC addresses this by occluding the defect and continuously withdrawing secretions. The device consists of an open-cell sponge attached to external vacuum suction via tube (**Fig. 2**). The sponge induces the formation of granulation tissue, while vacuum suction improves perfusion and removes secretions.[21] Small defects with well-perfused surrounding tissue and noncompartmentalized adjacent collections are amenable. VAC has some advantages over stent placement, allowing simultaneous closure of luminal defects, drainage of infectious foci, and granulation tissue formation in the wound cavity.[22] To place the device, a feeding tube is inserted intranasally and then orally exteriorized. A sponge, cut to a size smaller than the wound cavity, is fixed to the tip of the tube with suture. The sponge is grasped with endoscopic forceps and introduced into the fistula endoscopically. The feeding tube is then attached to continuous vacuum suction. The sponge is changed 2 or 3 times weekly. Ahrens and colleagues[23] reported its use for gastroesophageal anastomotic leaks. All 5 patients had leak closure at a median 42 days after a mean 9 sponge

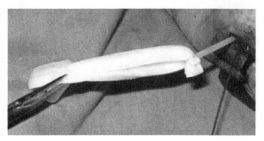

Fig. 1. Surgisis soft tissue graft attached to snare. (*Reprinted from* Tringali A, Daniel FB, Familiari P, et al. Endoscopic treatment of a recalcitrant esophageal fistula with new tools: stents, Surgisis, and nitinol staples (with video). Gastrointest Endosc 2010;72(3):647–50, Copyright from Elsevier; with permission.)

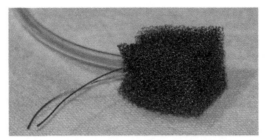

Fig. 2. Endoscopic vacuum-assisted sponge device. (*Reprinted from* Wedemeyer J, Brangewitz M, Kubicka S, et al. Management of major postsurgical gastroesophageal intrathoracic leaks with an endoscopic vacuum-assisted closure system. Gastrointest Endosc 2010;71(2):382–6, Copyright from Elsevier; with permission.)

changes. Two patients developed stenosis requiring dilation, and 1 patient had hemorrhage after dilation.

A cardiac septal occluder (Amplatzer Occluder; AGA Medical Corp., Plymouth, MN) has been used to close a postoperative esophagotracheal fistula after failure of endoscopic clip, glue, and stent therapy.[24] The device is a self-expanding nitinol wire mesh in the shape of 2 umbrellas linked together (**Fig. 3**). Under fluoroscopic and endoscopic guidance, a guidewire is inserted via the esophagus through the fistula and then orally exteriorized via the trachea. The occluder is then inserted on the guidewire and released first on the tracheal side and then on the esophageal side. Durable results were noted at 8 months.

BARIATRIC LEAKS AND FISTULAE
Scope of the Problem

Postoperative leaks have been reported in 1.7 to 5.2% of patients after Roux-en-Y gastric bypass (RYGB) and in 1.5% to 2.4% after sleeve gastrectomy (SG).[25–27]

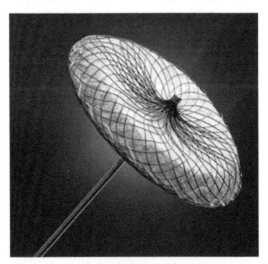

Fig. 3. Amplatzer cardiac septal occluder. (*Reprinted from* Repici A, Presbitero P, Carlino A, et al. First human case of esophgagus-tracheal fistula closure by using a cardiac septal occluder (with video). Gastrointestinal Endosc 2010;71(4):867–9, Copyright from Elsevier; with permission.)

Leak after RYGB can occur at the gastric pouch, gastrojejunal anastomosis, jejunal stump, jejunojejunal anastomosis, excluded stomach, duodenal stump (in resectional bypass), and blind jejunal limb.[28] Leaks most commonly occur at the gastrojejunal (68%) or jejunojejunal (5%) anastomosis, at the gastric pouch staple lines (10%), or at multiple sites (14%).[29] Leaks in the defunctionalized stomach may be especially challenging to diagnose. Most leaks in patients with SG occur in the proximal third of the stomach (85.7%).[30] Distal stenosis may predispose to fistula formation.[31] Leak is a major risk factor for mortality after bariatric surgery.[32] The mortality rate after leak is 6% to 14.7%, with a mortality rate of 9% after leak at the gastrojejunal anastomosis but 40% after leak at the jejunojejunal anastomosis.[33,34] After RYGB, chronic gastrogastric fistula occurs more commonly with the open approach, when the pouch is contiguous with the excluded stomach.[35]

Past Management Options

Management of postoperative leak is complicated by infection, multiorgan failure, and nutritional deficiency. Surgical management results in a high conversion rate to open surgery (48%), morbidity (up to 50%), and mortality (2%–10%).[36–40] Conservative management entails percutaneous drainage of collections, distal enteral or total parenteral feeding, and broad-spectrum antibiotics.

Current Status

Endoscopic techniques to address leak and fistula after bariatric surgery offer an excellent safety profile compared with surgical management. Endoscopic management should include dilation of distal stenoses if necessary. Closure can be performed with clips, sealants, and suturing devices. Stents can exclude defects to promote healing.

Leak source must be localized before therapy can be effectively performed. The procedure is started by performing a bubble test. The external drain is submerged underwater, and carbon dioxide is insufflated through the endoscope. The presence of bubbles indicates open communication with the drain. The next step is the injection of methylene blue with contrast into the drain with simultaneous endoscopic and fluoroscopic visualization of the suspected leak sites. Once the site is localized, the optimal therapy can be selected. If the leak is in the proximal pouch, a stent is the likely optimal therapy. If the leak is in a recessed area, such as the blind portion of the Roux limb, or in the distal bowel, a stent will not be effective; clips, sealants, or suturing should be considered.

Placement of both SEMS and SEPS for the treatment of leaks and fistulae is supported by considerable evidence. Enteral nutrition can be resumed during the healing process, and parenteral nutrition can be avoided. Extraluminal contamination is decreased, resulting in less infection and pain.[25] A meta-analysis of 7 studies of stent placement (including both SEMS and SEPS) for the treatment of acute leak after bariatric surgery found a pooled proportion for radiographic evidence of leak closure after stent removal of 87.8% (95% CI 79.4–94.2%).[41] Duration of stent therapy was between 4 and 8 weeks in most cases. Only 9% of patients proceeded to revision surgery. The pooled proportion of stent migration was 16.9% (95% CI 9.3–26.3%). Stent placement after SG has been shown effective in small case series.[42,43] Future bariatric-specific stent designs may improve efficacy and migration rate.

SEMS and SEPS each have advantages. SEPS are more likely to migrate. The use of partially covered SEMS decreases migration risk, but tissue ingrowth may complicate removal. In these cases, large-diameter SEPS placed within the SEMS can cause pressure necrosis of the ingrown tissue, and both stents can be removed together a few days later.[44] Alternatively, ingrown tissue can be fulgurated with argon plasma coagulation. Fully covered SEMS are effective for the treatment of leak and fistula, and migration can be prevented by securing the proximal end of the stent to the mucosa. Placement of 2 to 4 endoscopic clips on fully covered SEMS resulted in a migration rate of 13% versus 57% in the control group.[45] Attachment of a polypectomy snare to a stent, with the catheter exteriorized nasally and attached to the earlobe, has also been reported.[46]

Stents are placed using a forward-viewing endoscope and fluoroscopic visualization. The leak site and gastroesophageal junction should be marked externally using radio-opaque markers. The endoscope should be advanced into the Roux limb (in patients with RYGB) or the third portion of the duodenum (in patients with SG), and a guidewire should be introduced. The endoscope can then be removed and the stent delivery system inserted with fluoroscopic visualization. Stent length should be chosen so that the proximal end does not approach the upper esophageal sphincter (inducing globus sensation) and the distal end does not impact the enteral wall (inducing ulceration, bleeding, or perforation). A stiff guidewire can be used to assist traversal of acute angulation. Once the stent is deployed, its position can be adjusted endoscopically with forceps.

Sealants have shown efficacy in leak and fistula closure after bariatric surgery. The target mucosa should be ablated or excoriated to assist healing. A double-lumen catheter can be used to apply glue endoscopically, with the more viscous component inserted via the larger lumen (rapid-exchange catheters should not be used as they are prone to leakage). The fibrin is injected, forming a plug as it hardens. Fibrin sealant can also be used to fill residual cavities. Rábago and colleagues[47] studied fistula closure with fibrin in a series of 15 patients after failure of conservative therapy; 86.6% sealed after a mean 2.5 sessions. High-output fistulae were less likely to seal. Wong and colleagues[48] used a 5-mm choledochoscope to perform fistuloscopy in patients with postoperative gastrointestinal fistulae; fibrin glue was inserted, and some irrigation and debridement were concurrently performed in some patients. Nine of 9 fistulae were successfully sealed with no recurrence after 12 months. Cyanoacrylate, another sealant, is associated with tissue necrosis and inflammatory response; however, it is not inactivated by gastric or pancreatic enzymes.[49,50] It has shown efficacy in closure of fistulae in small series.[51]

Multimodality therapy is often required. Bége and colleagues[49] prospectively evaluated an entirely endoscopic approach for management of fistulae after bariatric surgery in 27 patients. Clips, cyanoacrylate glue, and stents were used alone or in combination, often after endoscopic debridement. The first procedure was successful in 41%, but all patients eventually achieved resolution after a mean 4.4 endoscopies at a mean 86 days. Lippert and colleagues[52] reported a success rate of 36.5% with fibrin alone and a 55.7% success rate with multimodal endoscopic therapy in a series of 52 patients with gastrointestinal fistula. Infection was a predictor of failure.

New Endoluminal Options

Surgisis AFP plugs (Cook Biotech, West Lafayette, IN), developed for surgical treatment of anal fistulae, have shown success in the treatment of enterocutaneous fistulae after bariatric surgery.[53] The acellular nature of Surgisis, a fibrogenic matrix, means that it can stimulate fistula closure without inducing an inflammatory foreign-body reaction.[54] Toussaint and colleagues[53] demonstrated closure of 4 of 5 enterocutaneous fistulae in 1 or 2 procedures. SEMS were used concurrently in some patients. Surgisis AFP insertion is performed under fluoroscopic guidance. The fistula tract is opacified with contrast, and a guidewire is inserted into the percutaneous fistula opening. The other end of the guidewire is captured with a snare and orally exterior-ized. The fistula tract is abraded over the guidewire. Next, a snare is passed through the fistula over the wire and used to grab the narrow end of the Surgisis plug. It is used to pull the plug into the fistula. Multiple plugs can be placed adjacently into a large-diameter fistula. Surgisis strips and AFP were used to treat gastrocutaneous fistulae in 25 post-RYGB patients.[55] The AFP (5 patients) were deployed into fistulae as described earlier; strips (20 patients) were maneuvered into the fistula from the luminal end using a polypectomy snare. Successful closure was achieved in all patients treated with AFP and 75% of patients treated with strips.

Endoscopic suturing techniques are effective for fistula closure (**Fig. 4**). However, device limitations and procedural complexity mean specialized technical skill is required. Fernandez-Esparrach and colleagues[56] used the Bard EndoCinch (CR Bard, Murray Hill, NJ) to repair gastrogastric fistulae. Although initial success was achieved in 95% of patients, the durable success rate was 35%. Fistulae with a diam-eter less than or equal to 10 mm had the best outcomes; no fistula with a diameter greater than 20 mm remained sealed. Inadequate suture placement depth may have been responsible for the lack of durable closure. One patient had significant bleeding, and another had esophageal perforation. The StomaphyX suturing system (EndoGastric Solutions, Redmond, WA) was used by Overcash[57] to repair 2 gastric leaks. One achieved a reduction of leak rate, and the other achieved leak resolution. The Apollo OverStitch (Apollo Endosurgery, Austin, TX), which creates full-thickness plications, achieved durable gastrogastric fistula closure in 3 of 7 cases in an abstract presented by Watson and Thompson.[58] There were no procedural complications.

COLONIC LEAKS AND FISTULAE
Scope of the Problem

Anastomotic leak after colonic surgery is the most serious postoperative complication. Colonic anastomosis leak rate has been reported as 3%, with mortality rates of 10.1%.[59] Postoperative leak should be suspected when fever, abdominal pain, sepsis, peritonitis, or fecal discharge from the drain or wound is present. C-reactive protein greater than 14 g/dL is a sensitive and specific marker for anastomotic leak.[60] Diag-nosis is often delayed, with a clinical diagnosis made at a median of 7 days and radio-logic diagnosis made at a median of 16 days; 42% are diagnosed after hospital discharge.[61]

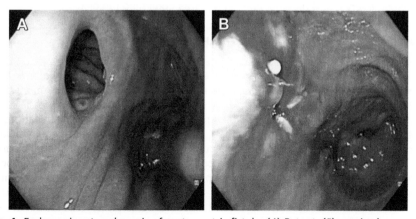

Fig. 4. Endoscopic sutured repair of gastrogastric fistula: (*A*) Patent, (*B*) repaired.

New Endoluminal Options

The endosponge method used in VAC can be applied to colonic anastomotic leaks.[62] The sponge is cut to the size and shape of the cavity that must be filled; a drainage tube with side ports is inserted into the sponge and secured with suture. An introducer sleeve is placed over the endoscope and advanced to the cavity. The sponge is inserted into the cavity, and the introducer sleeve is withdrawn. Vacuum is applied, and endoscopic visualization can ensure that the sponge is fully within the cavity. Multiple sponges are placed in series, and the sponge system is changed every 2 to 3 days. In 1 series, 28 of 29 patients had healing; hospital stays were long at a mean 34.4 days, and a mean 11.4 endoscopies were required. Another series found resolution of anastomotic leakage in 6 of 8 patients initiated at a median 24 days postoperatively and resolution in 3 of 8 patients initiated at a median 74 days after surgery.[63]

Stent placement has been reported for the treatment of anastomotic obstruction with leak presenting after colectomy with ileorectal anastomosis.[64] Dehiscence of approximately 40% of the anastomosis was noted, along with an associated abscess cavity. Using endoscopic and fluoroscopic guidance, a Polyflex stent (Boston Scientific, Natick, MA) was placed. Despite the use of clips to anchor the stent, the stent migrated and repeat stent placement was performed. Repeat endoscopy showed a healed anastomosis without stricture after 3 months.

OTSC has been used to successfully close postoperative anastomotic leaks after colonic resection, postoperative colonic fistulae, and colonic perforations after polypectomy. In 1 series, all 3 colonic fistulae recurred but all 4 colonic perforations were durably closed.[65] Another series reported successful closure of 2 of 3 postoperative fistulae (colorectal anastomosis and colocutaneous; failure of colovesical) and 1 successful closure of postoperative anastomotic dehiscence after left colectomy.[14] A series of OTSC closure of colorectal anastomosis, colocolic anastomosis, and 2 postoperative rectal fistulae reported durable closure in all cases.[15]

Endoscopic needle knife therapy with doxycycline injection has been used to treat a persistent 85 × 9-mm chronic sinus at the anastomosis after restorative proctocolectomy and ileal pouch-anal anastomosis.[66] The orifice of the sinus was opened with a triple-lumen needle knife (Olympus Medical Systems, Tokyo, Japan) and ERBE electrocautery (USA Incorporated Surgical Systems, Marietta, GA) with ERCP Endocut settings under Doppler ultrasound guidance. Doxycycline, 100 mg, IV solution powder dissolved in 10 mL normal saline was inserted into the sinus tract. Six sessions were performed every 2 to 3 months, and healing was confirmed radiologically.

PANCREATICOBILIARY LEAKS AND FISTULAE
Cholecystectomy

The incidence of major bile duct injury after laparoscopic cholecystectomy has recently been reported at 0.38%, and the rate of minor injury has been reported at 0.86%.[67] Minor injuries are usually defined as those of the cholecystohepatic duct (duct of Lushka), partial disruption of the right posterior sectoral duct, injuries to small subsegmental ducts in the gallbladder bed, and cystic duct stump leaks. Major biliary injuries are those of the common hepatic duct, common bile duct, right hepatic duct, and transection of the right posterior sectoral duct. Minor biliary injuries are typically managed endoscopically; however, major injuries may require surgical management.[68,69]

The rate of bile leak resolution after stent placement approaches 100%.[67] The leak does not need to be bridged. However, some controversies remain. Larger diameter stents are thought to improve drainage, but a randomized trial comparing 7-Fr and 10-Fr stents showed only a trend toward better drainage with larger diameters.[70] The role of sphincterotomy is controversial as well. Sphincterotomy can result in bleeding or perforation and is associated with an increase in complication rates of 7.3% to 9.8% and a mortality of up to 1.3%. However, it may decrease the incidence of post-ERCP pancreatitis. Sphincterotomy without stent insertion is inferior to stent placement alone.[71] It may be prudent to reserve sphincterotomy for cases complicated by cholangitis.

Distal Pancreatectomy

The incidence of postoperative pancreatic fistula after distal pancreatectomy remains 15%.[72] The mortality rate of pancreatic leakage after distal pancreatectomy has been reported at 12%.[73] Reoperation for surgical leak repair is associated with even higher mortality. Once accumulated collections have been drained, pancreatic fistula should be addressed with a bridging, transpapillary stent, as it is associated with better outcome (92% resolution if stent is bridging vs 50% if stent is adjacent to disruption, or 44% if stent is transpapillary).[74] In patients in whom bridging of the leak site is not possible, stent placement can still be attempted, but with a lower rate of success. In such patients, Seewald and colleagues[75] demonstrated successful closure of pancreatic fistula by the injection of cyanoacrylate glue into the fistula tract in 8 of 12 patients. They reported no procedure-related complications. The glue was mixed with Lipiodol (Ultra-Fluid; Guerbert GmbH, Sulzbach, Germany) contrast to allow fluoroscopic visualization. In additional, coil placement has been shown to be an effective alternative to treat leaks after distal pancreatectomy.[76] In a patient who had already failed pancreatic sphincterotomy and stent placement, a 0.035-in-diameter coil for intravascular use (Target Vascular, Boston Scientific, Cork, Ireland) was preloaded onto an ERCP catheter and deployed under fluoroscopic guidance. The leak closed within 3 weeks and remained closed 12 months later.

Hepatic Resection

The rate of biliary leakage after liver resection has been reported as 5.0% and is higher in patients with hepaticojejunostomy (13.6% vs 3.2%).[77] Septic complications and hepatic failure may result. Anastomotic leaks reportedly account for one-third of the postoperative mortality after major resective liver surgery.[78] Endoscopic stent placement is an option in patients without hepaticojejunostomy. ERCP and stent placement with and without biliary sphincterotomy was effective in posthepatectomy bile leak in 9 of 10 patients with polycystic liver disease.[79]

Hepatic Transplant

Bile leaks have been shown to occur in 5.0 to 13.3% of patients after hepatic transplant.[80,81] ERCP offers lower morbidity and mortality than surgery in the treatment of leak, and a higher success rate than percutaneous transhepatic cholangography drainage because of a lack of biliary dilation.[82] ERCP has been shown to locate leak site in 87.1% of cases and successfully treat the leak in 83.9%, although treatment of T-tube leak resulted in a higher rate of resolution (95.2%) than bridging stent treatment of anastomotic leak (42.9%).[83] Many anastomotic leaks progress to stricture despite treatment (73% in 1 series, most of which were successfully treated with stent placement).[81] Cystic duct stump leaks are often amenable to stent placement, whereas cut surface leaks are not. Placement of a nasobiliary drain allows constant suction drainage as well as repeat diagnostic cholangiography without ERCP.

SUMMARY

Postoperative leaks and fistulae are significant complications resulting in considerable morbidity and increased rate of mortality. Patients with these complications are likely already afflicted by infection, organ failure, and nutritional deficiency, and they are poor candidates for surgical revision. In additional, they present higher risk than the typical patient presenting for therapeutic endoscopy. Novel endoscopic therapies have demonstrated safety, despite the inherent challenges of intervention in this patient population, and are steadily building evidence for efficacy relative to surgical management.

REFERENCES

1. Rutegård M, Lagergren P, Rouvelas I, et al. Intrathoracic anastomotic leakage and mortality after esophageal cancer resection: a population-based study. Ann Surg Oncol 2012;19(1):99–103.
2. Alanezi K, Urschel JD. Mortality secondary to esophageal anastomotic leak. Ann Thorac Cardiovasc Surg 2004;10:71–5.
3. Lang H, Piso P, Stukenborg C, et al. Management and results of proximal anastomotic leak in a series of 1114 total gastrectomies for gastric carcinoma. Eur J Surg Oncol 2000;26:168–71.
4. Nowakowski P, Ziaja K, Ludyga T, et al. Self-expandable metallic stents in the treatment of post-esophagogastrostomy/post-esophagoenterostomy fistula. Dis Esophagus 2007;20:358–60.
5. Karl RC, Schreiber R, Boulware D, et al. Factors affecting morbidity, mortality, and survival in patients undergoing Ivor Lewis esophagogastrectomy. Ann Surg 2000; 231(5):635–43.
6. Noble F, Curtis N, Harris S, et al. Risk assessment using a novel score to predict anastomotic leak and major complications after oesophageal resection. J Gastrointest Surg 2012;16(6):1083–95.
7. Tsujimoto H, Ono S, Takahata R, et al. Systemic inflammatory response syndrome as a predictor of anastomotic leakage after esophagectomy. Surg Today 2012; 42(2):141–6.
8. Freeman RK, Ascioti AJ, Giannini T, et al. Analysis of unsuccessful esophageal stent placements for esophageal perforation, fistula, or anastomotic leak. Ann Thorac Surg 2012;94(3):959–65.
9. Černá M, Köcher M, Válek V, et al. Covered biodegradable stent: new therapeutic option for the management of esophageal perforation or anastomotic leak. Cardiovasc Intervent Radiol 2011;34(6):1267–71.
10. Han XW, Li YD, Wu G, et al. New covered mushroom-shaped metallic stent for managing anastomotic leak after esophagogastrostomy with a wide gastric tube. Ann Thorac Surg 2006;82(2):702–6.
11. Felsher J, Farres H, Chand B, et al. Mucosal apposition in endoscopic suturing. Gastrointest Endosc 2003;58(6):867–70.
12. Surace M, Mercky P, Demarquay JF, et al. Endoscopic management of GI fistulae with the over-the-scope clip system (with video). Gastrointest Endosc 2011;74(6): 1416–9.
13. von Renteln D, Denzer UW, Schachschal G, et al. Endoscopic closure of GI fistulae by using an over-the-scope clip (with videos). Gastrointest Endosc 2010;72(6):1289–96.
14. Parodi A, Repici A, Pedroni A, et al. Endoscopic management of GI perforations with a new over-the-scope clip device (with videos). Gastrointest Endosc 2010; 72(4):881–6.

15. Manta R, Manno M, Bertani H, et al. Endoscopic treatment of gastrointestinal fistulas using an over-the-scope clip (OTSC) device: case series from a tertiary referral center. Endoscopy 2011;43(6):545–8.
16. Pohl J, Borgulya M, Lorenz D, et al. Endoscopic closure of postoperative esophageal leaks with a novel over-the-scope clip system. Endoscopy 2010;42(9): 757–9.
17. Pramateftakis MG, Vrakas G, Kanellos I, et al. Endoscopic application of n-butyl-2-cyanoacrylate on esophagojejunal anastomotic leak: a case report. J Med Case Rep 2011;5:96.
18. Farra J, Zhuge Y, Neville HL, et al. Submucosal fibrin glue injection for closure of recurrent tracheoesophageal fistula. Pediatr Surg Int 2010;26(2):237–40.
19. Böhm G, Mossdorf A, Klink C, et al. Treatment algorithm for postoperative upper gastrointestinal fistulas and leaks using combined vicryl plug and fibrin glue. Endoscopy 2010;42(7):599–602.
20. Tringali A, Daniel FB, Familiari P, et al. Endoscopic treatment of a recalcitrant esophageal fistula with new tools: stents, Surgisis, and nitinol staples (with video). Gastrointest Endosc 2010;72(3):647–50.
21. Holle G, Riedel K, von Gregory H, et al. Vacuum-assisted closure therapy: current status and basic research. Unfallchirurg 2007;110:490–504 [in German].
22. Loske G, Schorsch T, Müller C. Endoscopic vacuum sponge therapy for esophageal defects. Surg Endosc 2010;24(10):2531–5.
23. Ahrens M, Schulte T, Egberts J, et al. Drainage of esophageal leakage using endoscopic vacuum therapy: a prospective pilot study. Endoscopy 2010;42(9): 693–8.
24. Repici A, Presbitero P, Carlino A, et al. First human case of esophagus-tracheal fistula closure by using a cardiac septal occluder (with video). Gastrointest Endosc 2010;71(4):867–9.
25. Morales MP, Miedema BW, Scott JS, et al. Management of postsurgical leaks in the bariatric patient. Gastrointest Endosc Clin N Am 2011;21(2):295–304.
26. Aurora AR, Khaitan L, Saber AA. Sleeve gastrectomy and the risk of leak: a systematic analysis of 4,888 patients. Surg Endosc 2012;26(6):1509–15.
27. Sakran N, Goitein D, Raziel A, et al. Gastric leaks after sleeve gastrectomy: a multicenter experience with 2,834 patients. Surg Endosc 2012. [Epub ahead of print].
28. Csendes A, Burgos AM, Braghetto I. Classification and management of leaks after gastric bypass for patients with morbid obesity: a prospective study of 60 patients. Obes Surg 2012;22(6):855–62.
29. Ballesta C, Berindoague R, Cabrera M, et al. Management of anastomotic leaks after laparoscopic Roux-en-Y gastric bypass. Obes Surg 2008;18:623–30.
30. Burgos AM, Braghetto I, Csendes A, et al. Gastric leak after laparoscopic-sleeve gastrectomy for obesity. Obes Surg 2009;19:1672–7.
31. Yehoshua RT, Eidelman LA, Stein M, et al. Laparoscopic sleeve gastrectomy—volume and pressure assessment. Obes Surg 2008;18(9):1083–8.
32. Almahmeed T, Gonzalez R, Nelson LG, et al. Morbidity of anastomotic leaks in patients undergoing Roux-en-Y gastric bypass. Arch Surg 2007;142(10):954–7.
33. Lee S, Carmody B, Wolfe L, et al. Effect of location and speed of diagnosis on anastomotic leak outcomes in 3828 gastric bypass cases. J Gastrointest Surg 2007;11(6):708–13.
34. Carucci LR, Turner MA, Conklin RC, et al. Roux-en-Y gastric bypass surgery for morbid obesity: evaluation of postoperative extraluminal leaks with upper gastrointestinal series. Radiology 2006;238(1):119–27.

35. MacLean LD, Rhode BM, Nohr C, et al. Stomal ulcer after gastric bypass. J Am Coll Surg 1997;185:1–7.
36. Gonzalez R, Sarr MG, Smith CD, et al. Diagnosis and contemporary management of anastomotic leaks after gastric bypass for obesity. J Am Coll Surg 2007;204(1): 47–55.
37. Madan AK, Martinez JM, Lo Menzo E, et al. Omental reinforcement for intraoperative leak repairs during laparoscopic Roux-en-Y gastric bypass. Am Surg 2009; 75(9):839–42.
38. Dapri G, Cadiere GB, Himpens J. Laparoscopic conversion of adjustable gastric banding and vertical banded gastroplasty to duodenal switch. Surg Obes Relat Dis 2009;5:678–83.
39. Ryou M, Ryan MB, Thompson CC. Current status of endoluminal bariatric procedures for primary and revision indications. Gastrointest Endosc Clin N Am 2011; 21(2):315–33.
40. Madan AK, Lanier B, Tichansky DS. Laparoscopic repair of gastrointestinal leaks after laparoscopic gastric bypass. Am Surg 2006;72(7):586–90.
41. Puli SR, Spofford IS, Thompson CC. Use of self-expandable stents in the treatment of bariatric surgery leaks: a systematic review and meta-analysis. Gastrointest Endosc 2012;75(2):287–93.
42. de Aretxabala X, Leon J, Wiedmaier G, et al. Gastric leak after sleeve gastrectomy: analysis of its management. Obes Surg 2011;21(8):1232–7.
43. Nguyen NT, Nguyen XM, Dholakia C. The use of endoscopic stent in management of leaks after sleeve gastrectomy. Obes Surg 2010;20(9):1289–92.
44. Eisendrath P, Cremer M, Himpens J, et al. Endotherapy including temporary stenting of fistulas of the upper gastrointestinal tract after laparoscopic bariatric surgery. Endoscopy 2007;39(7):625–30.
45. Vanbiervliet G, Filippi J, Karimdjee BS, et al. The role of clips in preventing migration of fully covered metallic esophageal stents: a pilot comparative study. Surg Endosc 2012;26(1):53–9.
46. Manes G, Corsi F, Pallotta S, et al. Fixation of a covered self-expandable metal stent by means of a polypectomy snare: an easy method to prevent stent migration. Dig Liver Dis 2008;40(9):791–3.
47. Rábago LR, Ventosa N, Castro JL, et al. Endoscopic treatment of postoperative fistulas resistant to conservative management using biological fibrin glue. Endoscopy 2002;34(8):632–8.
48. Wong SK, Lam YH, Lau JY, et al. Diagnostic and therapeutic fistuloscopy: an adjuvant management in postoperative fistulas and abscesses after upper gastrointestinal surgery. Endoscopy 2000;32(4):311–3.
49. Bège T, Emungania O, Vitton V, et al. An endoscopic strategy for management of anastomotic complications from bariatric surgery: a prospective study. Gastrointest Endosc 2011;73(2):238–44.
50. Herod EL. Cyanoacrylates in dentistry: a review of the literature. J Can Dent Assoc 1990;12(3):141–5.
51. Lee YC, Na HG, Suh JH, et al. Three cases of fistulae arising from gastrointestinal tract treated with endoscopic injection of Histoacryl. Endoscopy 2001;33(2):184–6.
52. Lippert E, Klebl FH, Schweller F, et al. Fibrin glue in the endoscopic treatment of fistulae and anastomotic leakages of the gastrointestinal tract. Int J Colorectal Dis 2011;26(3):303–11.
53. Toussaint E, Eisendrath P, Kwan V, et al. Endoscopic treatment of postoperative enterocutaneous fistulas after bariatric surgery with the use of a fistula plug: report of five cases. Endoscopy 2009;41(6):560–3.

54. Ansaloni L, Cambrini P, Catena F, et al. Immune response to small intestinal submucosa (surgisis) implant in humans: preliminary observations. J Invest Surg 2007;20:237–41.
55. Maluf-Filho F, Hondo F, Halwan B, et al. Endoscopic treatment of Roux-en-Y gastric bypass-related gastrocutaneous fistulas using a novel biomaterial. Surg Endosc 2009;23(7):1541–5.
56. Fernandez-Esparrach G, Lautz DB, Thompson CC. Endoscopic repair of gastro-gastric fistula after Roux-en-Y gastric bypass: a less-invasive approach. Surg Obes Relat Dis 2010;6(3):282–8.
57. Overcash WT. Natural orifice surgery (NOS) using StomaphyX for repair of gastric leaks after bariatric revisions. Obes Surg 2008;18(7):882–5.
58. Watson RR, Thompson CC. Applications of a novel endoscopic suturing device in the GI tract [abstract]. Gastrointest Endosc 2011;73(4):AB105.
59. Francone TD, Saleem A, Read TA, et al. Ultimate fate of the leaking intestinal anas-tomosis: does leak mean permanent stoma? J Gastrointest Surg 2010;14(6):987–92.
60. Almeida AB, Faria G, Moreira H, et al. Elevated serum C-reactive protein as a predictive factor for anastomotic leakage in colorectal surgery. Int J Surg 2012;10(2):87–91.
61. Hyman N, Manchester TL, Osler T, et al. Anastomotic leaks after intestinal anas-tomosis: it's later than you think. Ann Surg 2007;245(2):254–8.
62. Weidenhagen R, Gruetzner KU, Wiecken T, et al. Endoscopic vacuum-assisted closure of anastomotic leakage following anterior resection of the rectum: a new method. Surg Endosc 2008;22(8):1818–25.
63. van Koperen PJ, van Berge Henegouwen MI, Rosman C, et al. The Dutch multi-center experience of the endo-sponge treatment for anastomotic leakage after colorectal surgery. Surg Endosc 2009;23(6):1379–83.
64. Abbas MA. Endoscopic management of acute colorectal anastomotic complica-tions with temporary stent. JSLS 2009;13(3):420–4.
65. Kirschniak A, Subotova N, Zieker D, et al. The Over-The-Scope Clip (OTSC) for the treatment of gastrointestinal bleeding, perforations, and fistulas. Surg Endosc 2011;25(9):2901–5.
66. Li Y, Shen B. Successful endoscopic needle knife therapy combined with topical doxycycline injection of chronic sinus at ileal pouch-anal anastomosis. Colorectal Dis 2012;14(4):e197–9.
67. Karvonen J, Gullichsen R, Laine S, et al. Bile duct injuries during laparoscopic cholecystectomy: primary and long-term results from a single institution. Surg En-dosc 2007;21(7):1069–73.
68. Bergman JJ, van den Brink GR, Rauws EA, et al. Treatment of bile duct lesions after laparoscopic cholecystectomy. Gut 1996;38:141–7.
69. Schmidt SC, Langrehr JM, Hintze RE, et al. Long-term results and risk factors influencing outcome of major bile duct injuries following cholecystectomy. Br J Surg 2005;92:76–82.
70. Katsinelos P, Kountouras J, Paroutoglou G, et al. A comparative study of 10-Fr vs. 7-Fr straight plastic stents in the treatment of postcholecystectomy bile leak. Surg Endosc 2008;22(1):101–6.
71. Kaffes AJ, Hourigan L, De Luca N, et al. Impact of endoscopic intervention in 100 patients with suspected postcholecystectomy bile leak. Gastrointest Endosc 2005;61(2):269–75.
72. Hashimoto Y, Traverso LW. After distal pancreatectomy pancreatic leakage from the stump of the pancreas may be due to drain failure or pancreatic ductal back pressure. J Gastrointest Surg 2012;16(5):993–1003.

73. Adam U, Makowiec F, Riediger H, et al. Pancreatic leakage after pancreas resection. An analysis of 345 operated patients. Chirurg 2002;73(5):466–73 [in German].
74. Telford JJ, Farrell JJ, Saltzman JR, et al. Pancreatic stent placement for duct disruption. Gastrointest Endosc 2002;56(1):18–24.
75. Seewald S, Brand B, Groth S, et al. Endoscopic sealing of pancreatic fistula by using N-butyl-2-cyanoacrylate. Gastrointest Endosc 2004;59(4):463–70.
76. Lüthen R, Jaklin P, Cohnen M. Permanent closure of a pancreatic duct leak by endoscopic coiling. Endoscopy 2007;39(Suppl 1):E21–2.
77. Hoekstra LT, van Gulik TM, Gouma DJ, et al. Posthepatectomy bile leakage: how to manage. Dig Surg 2012;29(1):48–53.
78. Fragulidis G, Marinis A, Polydorou A, et al. Managing injuries of hepatic duct confluence variants after major hepatobiliary surgery: an algorithmic approach. World J Gastroenterol 2008;14(19):3049–53.
79. Coelho-Prabhu N, Nagorney DM, Baron TH, et al. ERCP for the treatment of bile leak after partial hepatectomy and fenestration for symptomatic polycystic liver disease. World J Gastroenterol 2012;18(28):3705–9.
80. Johnston TD, Reddy KS, Khan TT, et al. ERCP in the management of early versus late biliary leaks after liver transplantation. Int Surg 2006;91(5):301–5.
81. Gunawansa N, McCall JL, Holden A, et al. Biliary complications following orthotopic liver transplantation: a 10-year audit. HPB (Oxford) 2011;13(6):391–9.
82. Park JS, Kim MH, Lee SK, et al. Efficacy of endoscopic and percutaneous treatments for biliary complications after cadaveric and living donor liver transplantation. Gastrointest Endosc 2003;57:78–85.
83. Pfau PR, Kochman ML, Lewis JD, et al. Endoscopic management of postoperative biliary complications in orthotopic liver transplantation. Gastrointest Endosc 2000;52(1):55–63.

Endoscopic Resection of Large Colon Polyps

Tonya Kaltenbach, MD, MS*, Roy Soetikno, MD

KEYWORDS

- Colonoscopy • Advanced polypectomy • Endoscopic mucosal resection
- Endoscopic submucosal dissection • Neoplasm • Colorectal cancer

KEY POINTS

- Endoscopic resection is a safe and efficacious approach for large neoplasms, high-grade dysplasia, or mucosal carcinomas in the colon and rectum.
- Used according to its indications, it provides curative resection and obviates the higher morbidity, mortality, and cost associated with alternative surgical treatment.
- Proficiency in dynamic submucosal injection, use of a stiff snare and clipping are key components to resection, particularly for non-polypoid lesions.
- Specimen orientation and preparation is important for precise pathologic assessment and staging.
- Standardization and training of the basic principles and techniques to an entire team are necessary to disseminate the practice of endoscopic resection.

Wisdom is not the product of schooling but the lifelong attempt to acquire it.
—*Albert Einstein, To J. Dispentiere - March 24, 1954. AEA 59–495*

INTRODUCTION

Endoscopic resection is the preferred treatment method of large colorectal polyps.[1] Its safety and efficacy has been shown.[2] Used according to its indications, it provides curative resection and obviates the higher morbidity, mortality, and cost associated with alternative surgical treatment.[3,4] Unfortunately, at present, endoscopic resections of large colorectal polyps are not standard practice in the United States. The technique is not widely taught during training. One's ability to acquire the knowledge to safely and efficaciously perform such resection, therefore, often requires lifelong learning.[5]

Veterans Affairs Palo Alto, Stanford University, 3801 Miranda Avenue, GI-111, Palo Alto, CA 94304, USA
* Corresponding author.
E-mail address: endoresection@me.com

Gastrointest Endoscopy Clin N Am 23 (2013) 137–152
http://dx.doi.org/10.1016/j.giec.2012.10.005
1052-5157/13/$ – see front matter Published by Elsevier Inc.

giendo.theclinics.com

Standardization of the basic principles and techniques is necessary to optimize the widespread practice of endoscopic resection of large colorectal polyps in the United States. These principles include understanding the selection of the appropriate lesions, the techniques, and taking prophylactic steps for bleeding and perforation. The success of large resections requires knowledge and experience of endoscopists, pathologists, surgeons, and staff, along with adequate equipment and accessories. Herein, the authors describe the currently available technique and technology for endoscopic resection of large colorectal polyps.

PREPARATION
Indications

The endoscopic morphology of adenomas and early colorectal cancer are classified as polypoid and nonpolypoid types.[6,7] The polypoid type includes pedunculated (0-Ip) and sessile-shaped (0-Is) lesions, and the nonpolypoid type includes superficial elevated (0-IIa) and flat (0-IIb) (both grouped as flat) and depressed (0-IIc) morphology. The large type 0-IIa are termed lateral spreading tumor (LST). They include lesions with a smooth or granular/nodular surface. The smooth surface has been described as nongranular (LST-NG) and often contains multiple foci of high-grade dysplasia or slightly invasive carcinoma. The granular surface type (LST-G) is typically a villous adenoma; and if it harbors slightly invasive carcinoma, it is typically located in the most protruding granule.[8]

Understanding of the lesion morphology, in turn, aids in the treatment algorithm.[9] Standard polypectomy can be used to remove large polypoid lesions, particularly pedunculated, although prophylactic technique to prevent bleeding usually is required. Endoscopic mucosal resection (EMR), using the inject and cut technique, can remove the large nonpolypoid or sessile colorectal lesions.[10] In piecemeal EMR, we can target the area of most concerning pathology for en bloc resection, such as the nodule of LST-G type lesions. Endoscopic submucosal dissection (ESD) technique, which is intended to remove diseased mucosa by dissecting through the middle to deeper layers of the submucosa, can refine our ability to remove lesions that are difficult, if not impossible, to remove using mucosal resection technique or lesions with concern for multifocal dysplasia or invasion, such as LST-NG, that is difficult to predict endoscopically.[11,12]

Real-time colonoscopic assessment of the suspected histopathology and estimation of the depth of invasion of the colorectal lesion is also vital in treatment planning. Large lesions limited to the mucosa can undergo curative endoscopic resection. Lesions with a minimal or moderate likelihood to contain submucosal invasion can be treated with endoscopic resection for diagnostic and therapeutic purposes. Patients whose lesions are strongly suggestive of invasion should be referred directly to surgery after a confirmatory biopsy because endoscopic resection will expose them to an unnecessary higher risk of bleeding, perforation, recurrence, and metastasis.[13,14] It is appropriate, after assessment of the lesion, to reschedule patients for a dedicated resection procedure to ensure that there is an appropriate discussion of the risks and benefits with patients as well as to plan for the necessary equipment, time, and personnel for the procedure (**Box 1**).

Management of Anticoagulant and Antiplatelet Medications

At present, there is no specific anticoagulant and antiplatelet medication guideline for the removal of large colon polyps. Whenever possible, deferring elective resection procedures in patients who are on short-term antiplatelet or anticoagulation therapy usually is the preferred route. Otherwise, we generally follow the American Society of Gastrointestinal Endoscopy's (ASGE) guidelines for performing *standard* polypectomy,[15] which recommend no interruption of antiplatelet medications, such as aspirin

---

Box 1
Indications for colonoscopic mucosal resection and submucosal dissection

1. A team to perform the mucosal resection and/or submucosal dissection safely and efficaciously is available

2. The neoplasm's does not have feature of massive submucosal or advanced invasion

3. Endoscopic resection

   a. Mucosal resection

      i. Lesion (nonpolypoid or sessile) with adenomatous- or villous adenomatous–appearing mucosa requiring resection at the submucosa to ensure cure

      ii. If the lesion is suspected to contain high-grade dysplasia or slight submucosal invasion, endoscopic mucosal resection (EMR) is indicated provided that the lesion is within the scope of EMR technique for en bloc removal

   b. Submucosal dissection[a]

      i. Early carcinoma larger than 20 mm, which is difficult to resect en bloc by EMR. The lesion should have been evaluated by magnification colonoscopy or Endoscopic Ultrasound (EUS) and found to be likely to be cured by endoscopic resection

      ii. Adenoma with nonlifting sign

      iii. Residual lesion after EMR larger than 10 mm, which is difficult to resect by EMR

   c. Pathologic evaluation provided proof of cure

      i. Well-differentiated carcinoma (without poorly differentiation)

      ii. Without lymphatic or vascular invasion

      iii. High-grade dysplasia or intramucosal cancer, regardless of size (limit of involvement in the United States)

      iv. Minute submucosal invasion less than 1000 μm from the muscularis mucosa or, if the muscularis mucosa is absent, the depth of measurement is performed from the surface of the lesion (limit of involvement in Japan)

      v. Vertical and lateral margins are free from carcinoma

[a] Endoscopic submucosal dissection (ESD) indications for colorectal lesions as per Japan Gastroenterological Endoscopy Society's study of colorectal ESD.

---

or nonsteroidal antiinflammatory drugs, but discontinuation of platelet aggregation inhibitors, such as ticlopidine and clopidogrel, for 7 to 10 days, and anticoagulation agents, such as warfarin, for 5 days before the procedure. High-risk patients with atrial fibrillation and valvular disease should receive intravenous heparin up to 6 hours or low-molecular-weight heparin up to 24 hours before the procedure.

For the postresection management, we individualize the reinstitution of medical therapy, assessing both the thromboembolic and bleeding risk. After large polyp resection, we typically close the mucosal defects of nonpolypoid or sessile lesions with endoscopic clips and perform mechanical synching of the stalk of polypoid ones. We generally instruct patients to continue to take daily aspirin 81 mg and to resume clopidogrel and warfarin 10 days after the procedure. In patients who have a high thromboembolic risk, we resume the heparin infusion 6 hours after the procedure.

Equipment and Tools

We use endoscopes equipped with an auxiliary water jet, an adult high-definition colonoscope, with the accessory channel at the 5-o'clock position, for right colon lesions or a therapeutic gastroscope, with the accessory channel at the 7:30-o'clock position, for left-sided lesions to improve angulation (**Box 2**). We selectively use the translucent distal attachment device to stabilize the endoscope position for visualization and resection, particularly in lesions located behind folds or when performing ESD.[16] We prepare diluted indigo carmine (0.2%) (1 ampule of indigo carmine with 20 mL of water in a 60-mL syringe) and submucosal injectant (approximately 5 drops of indigo carmine in 10-mL normal saline syringes). We use a 25-gauge injection catheter and stiff snares (typically the 20-mm spiral snare [SD-230–20, Olympus America, Center Valley, Pennsylvania]) for resection and the 10-mm oval snare (SD-210–10, Olympus America, Center Valley, Pennsylvania) for the removal of the small areas of residual, increased fibrosis or tight angulations. We have clips (Resolution Clip, Boston Scientific, Natick, Massachusetts; Instinct Clip, Cook Medical Inc, Winston-Salem, NC, USA; QuikClip 2, Olympus America, Center Valley, Pennsylvania; and Over-the-scope Clip, Ovesco Endoscopy, Tubingen, Germany) as well as nylon loops (Olympus America) readily available. We use Endostat II Microvasive electrosurgical unit (Boston Scientific, Natick, MA) to provide a mixed current at 35 W for the right-sided lesion and 40 W for the left-sided lesions, or the ERBE electrosurgical generator (VIO 330D; ERBE USA Marietta, Georgia) using the fractionated cutting mode EndoCutQ at effect 3, cut duration 1, and cut interval 4 for snare resection. We use the argon plasma coagulation (APC) at 60 W, 1.0 L/min flow for ablation. We do not use the coagulation mode for snare resection.

PROCEDURE

We use a standardized endoscopic resection approach to safely and efficaciously remove large lesions, which includes lesion assessment; injecting and cutting EMR and ESD-universal (U) techniques; immediate reassessment and treatment of residual, histologic preparation and assessment; and surveillance.

Assessment

The appearance and border, particularly of a large nonpolypoid lesion, is closely examined using image-enhanced endoscopy to assess the histopathology, estimate

---

Box 2
Tools for colonoscopy with endoscopic mucosal resection

1. Adult colonoscope (right) or therapeutic upper (left sided) with auxiliary water jet
2. Carbon dioxide regulator
3. Electrocautery generator
4. Diluted simethicone in 60-mL syringe
5. Indigo carmine in 60-mL syringe
6. Injection needle (25 gauge)
7. Injectant (10-mL syringes of diluted indigo carmine and saline; tattoo agent)
8. Stiff snare: 2 types (large 20mm and small 10mm)
9. Biopsy forceps (cold and hot of standard cup size)
10. Endoscopic clips and loops
11. Argon plasma coagulator with straight catheter
12. Retrieval net
13. Pins and Styrofoam

the depth of invasion, and delineate the neoplastic borders.[17,18] Specifically, following the initial lesion inspection with white light, we then examine the mucosal surface and vascular pattern using Narrow band imaging (NBI)[19] and then spray indigo carmine directly onto the area of the lesion.[20]

RESECTION
Large Pedunculated Lesions

Pedunculated lesions may be removed by snare-loop polypectomy at the middle or upper stalk. En bloc resection is a key component to accurate pathologic staging to assess for the level of invasion. For giant polyps, the injection of 4 to 8 mL of 1:10 000 epinephrine into both the polyp head and stalk resulted in a dramatic polyp size reduction and higher en bloc resection rates.[21] Prophylactic ligation of the feeding blood vessel of the large or thick stalk, using either a nylon loop or clip, prevents immediate or delayed bleeding (**Fig. 1**).[22–25]

Large Sessile and Flat Lesions

Inject and cut colorectal EMR
Dynamic submucosal injection Submucosal injection is a key step of endoscopic resection techniques. Conventionally, during the injection process, the needle remains in a relatively fixed position in the submucosa during the fluid injection, and the lumen is insufflated to visualize the insertion point of the needle. A variety of injectants, including glycerol (a hypertonic solution consisting of 10% glycerol and 5% fructose in a normal saline solution) and colloid-based solutions, such as hydroxyethyl starch[26] or succinylated gelatin,[27] have been shown to sustain the submucosal bleb.

We successfully sustain a submucosal bleb using simple, low-cost, normal saline coupled with a modified injection technique, *dynamic submucosal injection* (**Fig. 2**).[28] We first plan the path of injection and envision the necessary movements of the needle catheter, endoscope tip deflection, and lumen air volume that will mold the bleb accordingly. We engage the catheter probe at our intended injection site, expose the needle by instructing "needle out" to our assistant, gently jab through the mucosa, and adjust the catheter position further in or out of the accessory channel according to the plane while instructing the assist to inject. Following visual confirmation with an elevation of the mucosa, the assistant injects rapidly and steadily while we concomitantly make subtle maneuvers to produce a localized submucosal bleb. Specifically, we slightly adjust the injection catheter position by pulling it back into the accessory channel, we deflect up with our endoscope tip into the direction of the lumen, and then we slightly suction the lumen—all to mold the bleb.

We inject with a 25-gauge sclerotherapy needle. The use of a mixture of indigo carmine and saline provides rapid visual feedback of the postresection depth and confirms the resection plane; blue indicates that the cut was at the submucosa level. Total injection volume has not been defined and varies according to the size of the lesion; our injection volumes generally range between 10 and 50 mL. Notably, we do not routinely use epinephrine in the injectate.

Snare resection We use a stiff snare, typically starting with the 20-mm spiral (SD-230 U-20, Olympus, Center Valley, Pennsylvania), and then the 10-mm spiral for small residual or nonlifting areas (SD-210 U-10, Olympus, Center Valley, Pennsylvania). We orient the lesion at the level of the accessory channel (typically the 5-o'clock position) and initiate the resection at the easiest plane, placing the snare around the lifted area of interest. We keep the lumen insufflated with air for the wall to be stretched to avoid capturing the muscularis propria. However, after we position our snare around the intended lesion,

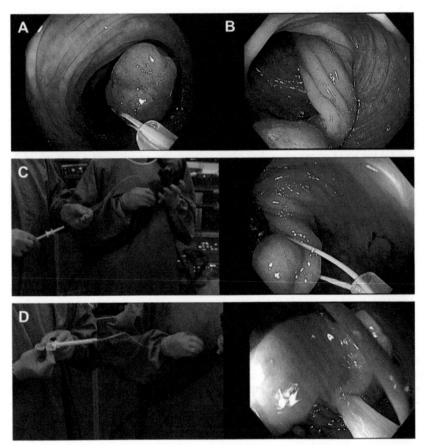

Fig. 1. Looping the stalk of a large pedunculated polyp to prevent bleeding. The essential aspects of endoscopic loop placement are to place the loop precisely at the base of the stalk and to recognize adequate closure. (*A, B*) This is optimal when the polyp is hanging and the colonoscope is positioned such that its channel is at the 6-o'clock position. (*C*) Use the sheath to close the loop, with the assistant using back-and-forth and to-and-fro motions of the yellow stopper of the sheath until the loop is maneuvered to the base of the stalk. (*D*) The snare should be closed tightly before application of current to prevent unintended burn at the area that has been strangulated by the loop because inadequate tightening of the snare may lead to the loop site having the smallest area and, thus, the highest current density.

we then slightly suction to collapse the distended colon and ease tissue capturing. The assistant slowly closes the snare until it is snug. We use a fulcrum position to provide more stiffness during the mucosal capture if the lesion cannot be easily captured into the snare (**Fig. 3**). Once the snare is closed tight, we then re-insufflate air to assess the amount of tissue captured. At this stage, before snare resection, we critically assess for muscularis propria entrapment. We instruct the assistant to slightly loosen the snare, and we deflect the endoscopic tip upward. Following the proper loosening step, we close the snare to the hub and resect the lesion. We repeat the injection and snare sequentially until there is no macroscopically visible lesion, being cognizant to avoid neoplastic bridges by placing one edge of the snare at the edge of the defect.

We perform various maneuvers during the procedure to complete the resection in a single session, such as manipulate the volume of air insufflation in the lumen,

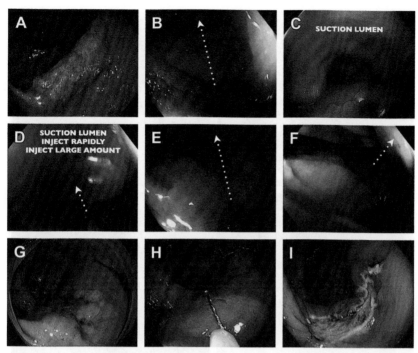

Fig. 2. Dynamic submucosal injection. (*A*) We first plan the flight path based on the lesion shape and location. (*B*) We engage the catheter probe at our intended injection site, expose the needle by instructing our assistant needle out, and adjust the catheter position further in or out of the accessory channel according to the plane while instructing the assist to inject. (*C*) The assistant injects rapidly and steadily a large amount of injectant while we concomitantly make subtle maneuvers to produce a localized submucosal bleb. The shape of the submucosal bleb is sculpted to provide a safe and effective resection. (*D*) The lumen was suctioned in order for the submucosal injectant to form a large bleb. (*E, F*) Further injection was performed at the distal side of the lesion. The tip of the endoscope was angulated up. (*F*) The tip of the endoscope was moved to the right. (*G*) After about 30 mL of submucosal injection. (*H*) A stiff snare was used to capture the lesion. The tip of the snare was impacted to the right side. The lumen was suctioned to bring the lesion into the snare. The lesion was cut in 2 parts. (*I*) The resection site with no residual neoplasms. Argon plasma coagulation was used to cauterize the edges and any visible microvessels on the resection surface. Arrows indicate (*B, D, E, F*) the intended direction of the endoscope tip and needle catheter during injection in order to optimize the submucosal bleb.

retroflex the endoscope to access lesions behind a fold, use a cap for stability, and change the snare size during the serial inject and cut resections, according to lesion position, location, and angle of approach (**Fig. 4**). We may also rotate the patient to optimize the polyp position or avoid the pooling of fluid or administer antispasmodic, such as glucagon 0.5 mg intravenously.

Reassessment

We aim to resect each lesion entirely during the initial session. The highest independent predictor of a failed complete endoscopic resection is a previous intervention (odds ratio 3.75, 95% confidence interval: 1.77–7.94; P = .001).[2] Residual tissue, in fact, leads to underlying fibrosis following electrocoagulation and, thus, nonlifting properties with subsequent submucosal injection, which can preclude complete resection. Thus, in our

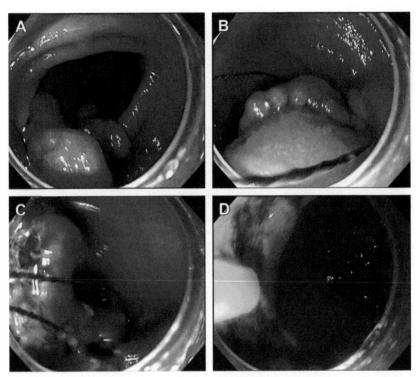

Fig. 3. Piecemeal EMR with fulcrum technique. (*A*) We used a distal translucent cap to optimize visualization and resection of the lesion that was overlying the folds. The angle remained difficult to direct the snare toward the correct plane of resection. (*B*) In such a case, we use the fulcrum technique to ensure that the snare was placed in a plane parallel to the fold. Following dynamic submucosal injection, the tip of the snare was impacted slightly to the right of the lesion. The snare was then slowly opened as the colonoscope was gently turned to the left. Close coordination between the endoscopist and assistant is required to perform this maneuver. The snare was pushed toward the lesion and air was suctioned slightly to draw the lesion into the snare. (*C*) The maneuver is repeated to allow resection of large pieces. (*D*) APC is used to ablate exposed superficial vessels and the resection edges.

practice, we remove any area of visible residual tissue. We apply APC to the bridges and periphery of the EMR defect sites. Following endoscopic treatment, we tattoo the sites of any lesion suspected of harboring invasive carcinoma.

ESD-U

Recent refinement of ESD instruments and skills has lead to its application in the treatment of large colorectal lesions as an alternative to EMR or surgery. The indications for colorectal ESD, however, are relatively few even at experienced centers because most colorectal neoplasms are benign and can be resected using piecemeal EMR with minimal risk of recurrence.[29]

ESD is generally accomplished using a variety of endoscopic knives and submucosal injectants. After generous submucosal injection, a marginal resection is performed to isolate the lesion with 3 or 4 mm surrounding normal mucosa. The submucosa under the lesion is injected further. With controlled movements, under direct view facilitated with the use of a cap, the ESD knife dissects through the submucosal layer to resect the

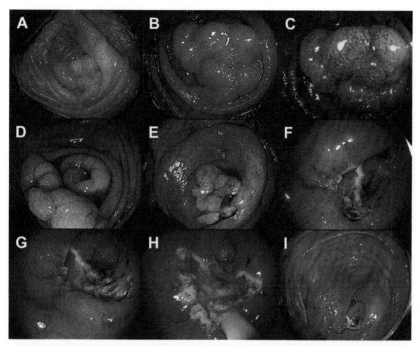

Fig. 4. EMR in difficult location at the periappendiceal orifice. (*A*) A lateral-spreading granular-type lesion can be seen in the cecum. Closer assessment using (*B*) high-definition white light, (*C*) narrow band imaging, and (*D*) indigo carmine show a villous surface pattern and that the lesion does not involve the appendix in its entirety. (*E*) Submucosal injection of diluted indigo carmine and normal saline shows partial lifting, which is typical of lesions near the appendiceal orifice in our experience. (*F*) A small oval 10-mm stiff snare is used to resect the lesion. (*G*) The blue hue of the stained submucosal resection defect can be easily seen. (*H*) The base and periphery are ablated using argon plasma coagulation. (*I*) More distant view of the cecum shows defect in relation to the appendiceal orifice. Pathology showed villous adenoma.

lesion in one piece. Several techniques have been described. Deliberate dissection of the submucosa under direct visualization permits lesions that otherwise cannot be captured by a snare or those with submucosa fibrosis to now be removed.

Although the current technique of ESD in the colon and rectum may pose some challenges, efforts are underway to simplify it toward less difficult, time-consuming, and risky techniques. The ESD with snaring method, (**Fig. 5**) described by Yamamoto and colleagues in 1999[30] and subsequently Toyonaga and colleagues in 2009,[31] uses the conventional snaring technique after circumferential incision. Toyonaga and colleagues also described the EMR with a small incision. In this technique, after submucosal injection, a small mucosal incision is made using the tip of the snare. Snaring can then be performed by engagement of the snare tip lightly into the incision. Fixing the tip of the snare, in turn, permits the opened snare to capture the surrounding normal mucosa of the lesion and prevent the snare from slipping. At present, the ESD with snaring and EMR with small incision techniques have been reported to lead to shorter procedure time, although data on their bleeding and complication rates are still limited.

Specimen Retrieval and Preparation

We retrieve (Roth net, US Endoscopy, Mentor, Ohio) the resected specimen intact for precise histologic processing. To maintain orientation of the specimen for pathologic

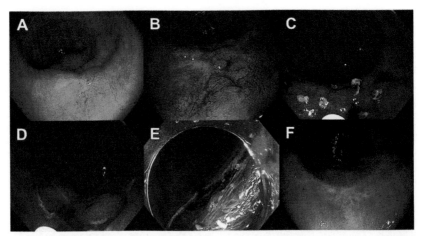

Fig. 5. ESD-U, ESD with snaring method in chronic ulcerative colitis. (*A*) The detection of dysplasia in long-standing ulcerative colitis can be difficult. (*B*) Indigo carmine was used to detect the dysplasia and determine the border of the flat lesion. It seemed to be benign. (*C*) Before submucosal injection, we marked the borders. (*D*) Followed by circumferential marginal incision. (*E*) After difficult en bloc snare resection, marked fibrosis can be appreciated. (*F*) Four-month surveillance showed no residual dysplasia.

fixation and prevent retraction and curling of the tissue, we insert fine pins at the periphery of the lesion and then gently stretch and fix it to a Styrofoam or wood plate. This preparation and 2-mm sectioning technique allows careful analysis of the histologic type, degree of differentiation, depth of vertical invasion, presence of ulceration, vessel involvement, and invasion of cancer into the resected margins. The resection can be diagnosed as complete when both the horizontal and vertical margins are negative.[32]

COMPLICATIONS OF ENDOSCOPIC RESECTIONS

Despite critical perceptions of EMR, skilled endoscopists have reported low adverse events. In comparison with the 20.1% morbidity and 1.3% mortality rates for surgery of colon tumors, general EMR data show a 0.7% to 3.7% for perforation and 0.4% to 3.8% for bleeding.[33] Indeed, the risks of EMR can be further decreased, and recent reported perforation rates of 1% remain too high. Based on our cumulative EMR data, we inform patients of a 1 in 150 rate of postresection bleeding (that can be treated with endoscopic hemostasis) and a theoretical risk of perforation. The key step to conquering the fear of complications is to practice the steps to prevent them and become proficient in the methods to treat them.

PREVENTING AND TREATING COMPLICATIONS
Bleeding

Bleeding can occur during or after resection. Immediate bleeding occurs when submucosal vessels are cut but insufficiently coagulated. Delayed bleeding arises when injured or coagulated vessels subsequently rupture. It is reported in approximately 7% of cases, is more clinically significant, and typically occurs within 48 hours after resection. The strategy to minimize the risks of bleeding includes the following: (1) use an appropriate assessment technique to avoid transecting into invasive cancers; (2) use an adequate submucosal injection to avoid transecting or injuring the deeper and larger submucosal vessels; (3) obliterate exposed postresection vessels using coagulation or endoscopic clips; and (4) prophylactically strangulate the feeding vessels of the pedunculated neoplasms. Ensuring that patients have adequate coagulation and clotting functions and being prepared to treat bleeding cannot be overemphasized. Routine prophylactic therapy for high-risk lesions, such as those on the right side, in the elderly, or in patients on antiplatelet agents, is yet defined.[34,35]

Perforation

Perforation can occur during or after resection. Immediate perforation occurs because of deep resection, whereas delayed perforation occurs from a rupture of the wall caused by coagulation necrosis. Our strategy prevent perforation includes the following: (1) use of an adequate amount of submucosal injection and recognizing the nonlifting sign; (2) lift the snare away into the lumen prior and slightly loosen it before complete snare resection to avoid entrapment of the muscularis propria; (3) immediately close frank perforation, suspected perforation, or any thin or excessively coagulated postresection sites; (**Fig. 6**) and (4) avoid performing too many large mucosal resections at the same session.

Each lesion is closely observed during and after submucosal injection to assess for the nonlifting sign to minimize the risk for a transmural burn or perforation and assess for submucosal invasion. Nonlifting may occur because the lesion contains carcinoma that has invaded the deeper part of the submucosa or the muscularis propria or because of prior multiple biopsies or resection attempts. The snare may inadvertently capture the muscularis propria at the area that does not lift and lead to subsequent perforation. As such, if patients are to be subsequently referred for mucosal resection, we recommend that biopsy should be deferred or limited to one site.

Endoscopic clips are particularly useful in the prevention or immediate treatment of perforation. Its successful use has been reported in prior studies.[36] We use the

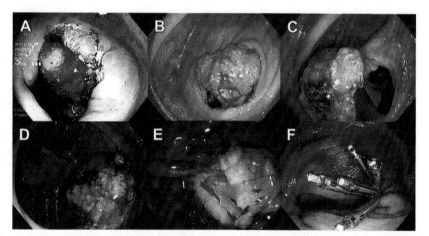

Fig. 6. Recognition and closure of postresection perforation. The most technically difficult endoscopic resection is one that has a prior incomplete resection. (*A*) This large sessile lesion was incompletely cut. The image was taken at the conclusion of the initial incomplete resection. (*B*) Two months later, the lesion seemed larger with convergence of folds at the scarred area. (*C*) The lesion at the opposite wall of the ileocecal valve is injected. (*D*) It partially lifted. (*E*) After snare resection, there is a 1-mm central defect. (*F*) Immediately, air was suctioned to decrease intraluminal pressure, carbon dioxide was used, and the defect was completely closed using multiple clips.

clipping method as a means to immediately suture suspicious or frank of perforation or areas deemed to be too thin or to have been excessively coagulated. We use carbon dioxide and deflate the colon immediately after performing large mucosal resection to decrease colonic pressure. Because the risk of bacterial seeding is not known, we also prescribe broad-spectrum antibiotics to be taken for 3 days.

Postoperative Care

We routinely discharge patients from our endoscopy unit after the resection of large colorectal polyps. We advise them to stay on a clear-liquid diet for the evening and to resume a regular diet as tolerated the following day.

REPORTING, FOLLOW-UP, AND CLINICAL IMPLICATIONS
Surveillance Colonoscopy

We perform surveillance colonoscopy at 6 months to assess for local recurrence in patients who underwent piecemeal EMR. On surveillance colonoscopy, we locate the prior EMR site based by a scar or tattoo. We inspect the innominate groove pattern closely to macroscopically assess for local recurrence using both high-definition, electronic-based, image-enhanced endoscopy and diluted indigo carmine. Repeat EMR is performed for local recurrence. Biopsies are obtained of the scarred site of lesions with advanced pathology if there is no macroscopic evidence of recurrence. In general, after a clearing examination, we repeat the examination at 1 and 3 years, although patients with giant lesions may undergo 3 successive yearly examinations. However, optimal surveillance intervals following resection of large colorectal polyps are not yet known.[37] We refer patients with submucosal invasive carcinoma or lesions not amenable to curative EMR for surgical resection.

CLINICAL OUTCOMES OF ENDOSCOPIC RESECTION

Numerous studies have shown the safe and effective endoscopic removal of large colorectal lesions,[2,38–44] although most large colorectal lesions continue to be referred for surgical resection.[45] Practitioners maintain that endoscopic resection cannot be generalized and that long-term efficacy and cost data are limited. However, in reality, the continued widespread surgical practice for benign colon lesions is likely caused by insufficient technical skills, perceived high complication risk, increased utilization of endoscopy resources and time, and inadequate reimbursement.[4,46] Without a proper reimbursement rate, it is likely that EMR will continue to be of limited availability.

Data from our referral cohort of 240 nonpolypoid lesions with a mean size of 24.5 ± 12.0 mm (range 10–80 mm) showed that we obviated surgery in 86.7% of the patients. One-third of the referred cohort had a previously attempted incomplete resection. Non-lifting properties (n = 20) were the main reason for surgical referral.[3] Others have published recurrence rates ranging from 0% to 40% following piecemeal endoscopic resection of large colorectal lesions. A recent series of approximately 300 polyps larger than 3 cm that were resected endoscopically demonstrated a recurrence rate of 17%, with most of the recurrent lesions successfully treated endoscopically.[47–49]

Notably, local recurrence refers to neoplasia, and not cancer; moreover, most local recurrence is successfully treated with endoscopy. Thus, local recurrence does not indicate endoscopic treatment failure, but rather serves to remind us of the importance of appropriate postresection surveillance and retreatment. In cases with residual neoplasia, appropriate therapy with biopsy or repeat EMR is prudent; another surveillance colonoscopy should be performed at 6 months. Subsequent examinations should be performed for 3 to 6 months until long-term eradication is confirmed, and then patients should resume surveillance at the recommended guideline inter-vals.[50] Khashab and colleagues[51] reported a high predictive value for long-term erad-ication in cases when the postmucosectomy scar site showed both normal macroscopic and microscopic (biopsy) findings.[52]

The results of colorectal ESD performed by expert endoscopists are promising. Saito and colleagues[53] reported the performance of ESD to remove 200 colorectal lesions that measured an average of 38 mm. In a median resection time of 90 minutes, they were able to obtain an en bloc resection rate of 84% and a curative resection of 83%. They had a 5% perforation rate, which they successfully treated by endoscopic clipping, except in 1 case (0.5%). Delayed bleeding occurred within the 5 days after the procedure. Others have reported similar data showing a high rate of en bloc resection and the ability to conservatively manage perforation with clipping, bowel rest, and antibiotics.[54]

The technical complexities of ESD in the colon have, nonetheless, precluded its widespread application in Western countries for the resection of large polyps. In addi-tion, truly nongranular flat lesions that would require ESD are quite uncommon. Thus, ESD in Western countries is rarely available.

CURRENT CONTROVERSIES/FUTURE CONSIDERATIONS

Endoscopic resection of large colorectal polyps can be safe and efficacious. Realisti-cally, however, the widespread adaptation of EMR and ESD techniques will require major shifts in training and practice culture. In the United States, for example, most patients who are diagnosed with large colon polyps are directly referred for surgery without an evaluation by an expert in endoscopic resection. This convention reflects the current lack of standardization and accountability in endoscopic knowledge, training, and practice. Moreover, it is driven by a variety of reasons, including insuffi-cient skill acquisition and competency, apprehension of higher complication risks, and reluctance to commit more endoscopic resources and time without adequate reim-bursement despite existing safety, efficacy, and cost-effectiveness data.

SUMMARY

Endoscopic resection is a safe and efficacious approach for large neoplasms, high-grade dysplasia, or mucosal carcinomas in the colon and rectum. Used according to its indications, it provides curative resection and obviates the higher morbidity, mortality, and cost associated with alternative surgical treatment.

REFERENCES

1. Soetikno R, Gotoda T. Con: colonoscopic resection of large neoplastic lesions is appropriate and safe. Am J Gastroenterol 2009;104:272–5.
2. Moss A, Bourke MJ, Williams SJ, et al. Endoscopic mucosal resection outcomes and prediction of submucosal cancer from advanced colonic mucosal neoplasia. Gastroenterology 2011;140:1909–18.
3. Kaltenbach T, Binmoeller K, Kalindindi V, et al. Endoscopic resection of large colorectal lesions in the United States in a referral center is a dominant strategy - long-term efficacy and cost analysis results. Am J Gastroenterol 2008;103:S169–206.
4. Swan MP, Bourke MJ, Alexander S, et al. Large refractory colonic polyps: is it time to change our practice? A prospective study of the clinical and economic impact of a tertiary referral colonic mucosal resection and polypectomy service (with videos). Gastrointest Endosc 2009;70:1128–36.

5. Kaltenbach T, Soetikno R, Kusano C, et al. Development of expertise in endoscopic mucosal resection and endoscopic submucosal dissection. Tech Gastrointest Endosc 2011;13:100–4.

6. Yasutomi M, Baba S, Hojo K, et al. Japanese classification of colorectal carcinoma. Tokyo (Japan): Kanehara & Co; 1997.

7. The Paris endoscopic classification of superficial neoplastic lesions: esophagus, stomach and colon. Gastrointest Endosc 2003;58:S3–43.

8. Sano Y, Iwadate M. The importance of the macroscopic classification of colorectal neoplasms. Gastrointest Endosc Clin N Am 2010;20:461–9.

9. Soetikno RM, Kaltenbach T, Rouse RV, et al. Prevalence of nonpolypoid (flat and depressed) colorectal neoplasms in asymptomatic and symptomatic adults. JAMA 2008;299:1027–35.

10. Soetikno RM, Gotoda T, Nakanishi Y, et al. Endoscopic mucosal resection. Gastrointest Endosc 2003;57:567–79.

11. Saito Y, Fujii T, Kondo H, et al. Endoscopic treatment for laterally spreading tumors in the colon. Endoscopy 2001;33:682–6.

12. Uraoka T, Saito Y, Matsuda T, et al. Endoscopic indications for endoscopic mucosal resection of laterally spreading tumours in the colorectum. Gut 2006; 55:1592–7.

13. Kaltenbach TS, Tada K, Saito Y, et al. Incidence of lymph node metastasis from sessile or nonpolypoid early colon cancer: stratified criteria when to operate or when to watch. Gastrointest Endosc 2011;73:AB291–2.

14. Kitajima K, Fujimori T, Fujii S, et al. Correlations between lymph node metastasis and depth of submucosal invasion in submucosal invasive colorectal carcinoma: a Japanese collaborative study. J Gastroenterol 2004;39:534–43.

15. Anderson MA, Ben-Menachem T, Gan SI, et al. Management of antithrombotic agents for endoscopic procedures. Gastrointest Endosc 2009;70:1060–70.

16. Sanchez-Yague A, Kaltenbach T, Yamamoto H, et al. The endoscopic cap that can (with videos). Gastrointest Endosc 2012;76:169–78.e1–2.

17. Kaltenbach T, Sano Y, Friedland S, et al. American Gastroenterological Association (AGA) Institute technology assessment on image-enhanced endoscopy. Gastroenterology 2008;134:327–40.

18. Kaltenbach T, Soetikno R. Image-enhanced endoscopy is critical in the detection, diagnosis, and treatment of non-polypoid colorectal neoplasms. Gastrointest Endosc Clin N Am 2010;20:471–85.

19. Hewett DG, Kaltenbach T, Sano Y, et al. Validation of a simple classification system for endoscopic diagnosis of small colorectal polyps using narrow-band imaging. Gastroenterology 2012;143:599–607.e1.

20. Kudo S, Hirota S, Nakajima T, et al. Colorectal tumours and pit pattern. J Clin Pathol 1994;47:880–5.

21. Hogan RB, Hogan RB 3rd. Epinephrine volume reduction of giant colon polyps facilitates endoscopic assessment and removal. Gastrointest Endosc 2007;66: 1018–22.

22. Hachisu T. A new detachable snare for hemostasis in the removal of large polyps or other elevated lesions. Surg Endosc 1991;5:70–4.

23. Iishi H, Tatsuta M, Narahara H, et al. Endoscopic resection of large pedunculated colorectal polyps using a detachable snare. Gastrointest Endosc 1996;44:594–7.

24. Kouklakis G, Mpoumponaris A, Gatopoulou A, et al. Endoscopic resection of large pedunculated colonic polyps and risk of postpolypectomy bleeding with adrenaline injection versus endoloop and hemoclip: a prospective, randomized study. Surg Endosc 2009;23:2732–7.

25. Di Giorgio P, De Luca L, Calcagno G, et al. Detachable snare versus epinephrine injection in the prevention of postpolypectomy bleeding: a randomized and controlled study. Endoscopy 2004;36:860–3.
26. Arezzo A, Pagano N, Romeo F, et al. Hydroxy-propyl-methyl-cellulose is a safe and effective lifting agent for endoscopic mucosal resection of large colorectal polyps. Surg Endosc 2009;23:1065–9.
27. Moss A, Bourke MJ, Metz AJ. A randomized, double-blind trial of succinylated gelatin submucosal injection for endoscopic resection of large sessile polyps of the colon. Am J Gastroenterol 2010;105:2375–82.
28. Soetikno R, Kaltenbach T. Dynamic submucosal injection technique. Gastrointest Endosc Clin N Am 2010;20:497–502.
29. Tanaka S, Tamegai Y, Tsuda S, et al. Multicenter questionnaire survey on the current situation of colorectal endoscopic submucosal dissection in Japan. Dig Endosc 2010;22(Suppl 1):S2–8.
30. Yamamoto H, Koiwai H, Yube T, et al. A successful single-step endoscopic resection of a 40 millimeter flat-elevated tumor in the rectum: endoscopic mucosal resection using sodium hyaluronate. Gastrointest Endosc 1999;50:701–4.
31. Toyonaga T, Man-I M, Morita Y, et al. The new resources of treatment for early stage colorectal tumors: EMR with small incision and simplified endoscopic submucosal dissection. Dig Endosc 2009;21:S31–7.
32. Mojtahed A, Shimoda T. Proper pathologic preparation and assessment of endoscopic mucosal resection and endoscopic submucosal dissection specimens. Tech Gastrointest Endosc 2011;13:95–9.
33. Clinical Outcomes of Surgical Therapy Study Group. A comparison of laparoscopically assisted and open colectomy for colon cancer. N Engl J Med 2004;350:2050–9.
34. Buddingh KT, Herngreen T, Haringsma J, et al. Location in the right hemi-colon is an independent risk factor for delayed post-polypectomy hemorrhage: a multi-center case-control study. Am J Gastroenterol 2011;106:1119–24.
35. Metz AJ, Bourke MJ, Moss A, et al. Factors that predict bleeding following endoscopic mucosal resection of large colonic lesions. Endoscopy 2011;43:506–11.
36. Raju GS, Saito Y, Matsuda T, et al. Endoscopic management of colonoscopic perforations (with videos). Gastrointest Endosc 2011;74:1380–8.
37. Lieberman DA, Rex DK, Winawer SJ, et al. Guidelines for colonoscopy surveillance after screening and polypectomy: a consensus update by the US Multi-Society Task Force on Colorectal Cancer. Gastroenterology 2012;143:844–57.
38. Kanamori T, Itoh M, Yokoyama Y, et al. Injection-incision-assisted snare resection of large sessile colorectal polyp. Gastrointest Endosc 1996;43:189–95.
39. Tanaka S, Haruma K, Oka S, et al. Clinicopathologic features and endoscopic treatment of superficially spreading colorectal neoplasms larger than 20 mm. Gastrointest Endosc 2001;54:62–6.
40. Su MY, Hsu CM, Ho YP, et al. Endoscopic mucosal resection for colonic non-polypoid neoplasms. Am J Gastroenterol 2005;100:2174–9.
41. Bergmann U, Beger HG. Endoscopic mucosal resection for advanced non-polypoid colorectal adenoma and early stage carcinoma. Surg Endosc 2003;17:475–9.
42. Arebi N, Swain D, Suzuki N, et al. Endoscopic mucosal resection of 161 cases of large sessile or flat colorectal polyps. Scand J Gastroenterol 2007;42:859–66.
43. Luigiano C, Consolo P, Scaffidi MG, et al. Endoscopic mucosal resection for large and giant sessile and flat colorectal polyps: a single-center experience with long-term follow-up. Endoscopy 2009;41:829–35.

44. Regula J, Wronska E, Polkowski M, et al. Argon plasma coagulation after piece-meal polypectomy of sessile colorectal adenomas: long-term follow-up study. Endoscopy 2003;35:212–8.
45. Onken JE, Friedman JY, Subramanian S, et al. Treatment patterns and costs associated with sessile colorectal polyps. Am J Gastroenterol 2002;97:2896–901.
46. Overhiser AJ, Rex DK. Work and resources needed for endoscopic resection of large sessile colorectal polyps. Clin Gastroenterol Hepatol 2007;5:1076–9.
47. Brooker JC, Saunders BP, Shah SG, et al. Treatment with argon plasma coagula-tion reduces recurrence after piecemeal resection of large sessile colonic polyps: a randomized trial and recommendations. Gastrointest Endosc 2002;55:371–5.
48. Iishi H, Tatsuta M, Iseki K, et al. Endoscopic piecemeal resection with submu-cosal saline injection of large sessile colorectal polyps. Gastrointest Endosc 2000;51:697–700.
49. Seitz U, Bohnacker S, Seewald S, et al. Long-term results of endoscopic removal of large colorectal adenomas. Endoscopy 2003;35:S41–4.
50. Winawer SJ, Zauber AG, Fletcher RH, et al. Guidelines for colonoscopy surveil-lance after polypectomy: a consensus update by the US Multi-Society Task Force on Colorectal Cancer and the American Cancer Society. Gastroenterology 2006; 130:1872–85.
51. Khashab M, Eid E, Rusche M, et al. Incidence and predictors of "late" recur-rences after endoscopic piecemeal resection of large sessile adenomas. Gastro-intest Endosc 2009;70:344–9.
52. Rose J, Schneider C, Yildirim C, et al. Complications in laparoscopic colorectal surgery: results of a multicentre trial. Tech Coloproctol 2004;8(Suppl 1):s25–8.
53. Saito Y, Uraoka T, Matsuda T, et al. Endoscopic treatment of large superficial colorectal tumors: a case series of 200 endoscopic submucosal dissections (with video). Gastrointest Endosc 2007;66:966–73.
54. Tamegai Y, Saito Y, Masaki N, et al. Endoscopic submucosal dissection: a safe technique for colorectal tumors. Endoscopy 2007;39:418–22.

Enteral Stents in Malignant Bowel Obstruction

A. Aziz Aadam, MD[a], John A. Martin, MD[b],*

KEYWORDS

- Malignant bowel obstruction • Self-expanding metal stent • Gastroduodenal stent
- Colonic stent

KEY POINTS

- Colorectal stent placement offers a minimally invasive approach for relief of malignant bowel obstruction.
- Stent placement is safe and effective in carefully selected patients as a bridge to surgery or for definitive palliation of obstruction.
- Concerns remain regarding the long-term efficacy of stent placement and related complications.
- Future studies are needed to identify patients who are the best candidates for stent placement.

INTRODUCTION

The role of endoscopy in malignant bowel obstruction has evolved rapidly over the past 2 decades. Self-expanding metal stents (SEMS) allow for the restoration of luminal patency and relief of obstructive symptoms. Surgery was previously the mainstay of treatment for malignant obstruction of the gastrointestinal tract, but endoscopic stent placement offers an effective therapeutic alternative. This review discusses the role of enteral stents in malignant gastroduodenal and colorectal obstruction. Stenting of the esophagus is discussed separately in an article elsewhere in this issue by Enestvedt and Ginsberg.

TECHNOLOGY

Dohmoto and colleagues[1] first described the use of an endoluminal prosthesis using a rigid Celestin tube for the palliation of rectal cancer. In 1992, Spinelli and colleagues[2]

a Medicine-Gastroenterology and Hepatology, Northwestern University, 675 N St Clair, Galter 17-250, Chicago, IL 60611; b Medicine-Gastroenterology and Hepatology and Surgery-Organ Transplantation, Director of Endoscopy, Northwestern University, 675 N St Clair, Galter 17-250, Chicago, IL 60611
* Corresponding author.
E-mail address: j-martin3@northwestern.edu

Gastrointest Endoscopy Clin N Am 23 (2013) 153–164
http://dx.doi.org/10.1016/j.giec.2012.10.006
1052-5157/13/$ – see front matter © 2013 Published by Elsevier Inc.

giendo.theclinics.com

reported palliation of malignant rectal obstruction in 4 patients by using a modified Gianturco-Rosch stent composed of stainless steel. In the past 20 years various SEMS have been developed, utilizing various metal alloys including stainless steel, Elgiloy, and nitinol. Nitinol is a nickel-titanium alloy and has largely replaced stainless steel and Elgiloy in the composition of SEMS. Nitinol offers superior flexibility and is also compatible with magnetic resonance imaging, but offers less radial force compared with SEMS made of other materials. The thermal properties of nitinol allow SEMS to fully expand to their maximum diameter at body temperature.[3]

SEMS exert self-expandable radial force owing to their unique metallic properties, and become anchored at the site of luminal obstruction. SEMS are available in various diameters and lengths, and differ in their delivery mechanisms. The efficacy of SEMS is limited by the potential for tumor ingrowth and overgrowth, migration, and luminal occlusions, as well as misdeployment and technical malfunctions. SEMS can be partially or wholly covered with a silicone membrane to prevent tumor penetration into the meshwork of the stent. However, currently available enteral stents in the United States are uncovered. The commercially available enteral stents in the United States are listed in **Table 1**.

Table 1
Commercially available enteral stents in the United States

	Stent			Delivery System		
	Diameter (mm)		Expanded		Catheter	Working
	Flare	Body	Length (cm)	Type	Diameter	Length (cm)
Boston Scientific						
Wallflex duodenal	27	22	6	TTS	10F	230
			9			
			12			
Wallflex colonic	30	25	6	TTS	10F	135
	27	22	9			
			12			230
Wallstent duodenal and	N/A	20	6	TTS	10F	160
colonic		22	9			255
			12			
Ultraflex colonic	30	25	5.7	OTW	22F	100
			8.7			
			11.7			
Cook Medical						
Evolution duodenal	27	22	6	TTS	10F	230
			9			
			12			
Evolution colonic	30	25	6	TTS	10F	230
			8			
			10			
Colonic Z-stent	35	25	4	OTW	10.3 mm	40
			6			
			8			
			12			

Abbreviations: N/A, no data available; OTW, over the wire; TTS, through the scope.

TECHNIQUE

The first step in the placement of an enteral stent is assessment of the malignant stricture (**Fig. 1**). Preprocedure cross-sectional imaging or, in certain instances, contrast studies, is helpful in determining the length and diameter of the stricture and degree of obstruction. During endoscopy the proximal extent of the stricture is identified. Gentle advancement of the endoscope through the stricture can be attempted, and is helpful in determining the length of the stricture. In the case of a nontraversable stricture, its length can be determined fluoroscopically with contrast injection. A guide wire is then advanced through the endoscope and placed well beyond the distal end of the stricture under fluoroscopic guidance (**Fig. 2**). Stricture length is determined even more precisely with the use of a balloon-tipped catheter; the balloon is inflated at the distal to the extent of the stricture, then pulled back toward the tip of the endoscope until resistance is palpable. Fluoroscopic visualization will then demonstrate the distance between the proximal end of the stricture nearest the endoscope tip, and the distal end of the stricture at the proximal end of the balloon. The stent selected should be 4 to 6 cm longer than the axial length of the stricture to adequately bridge the obstruction.

The two methods for stent deployment are the through-the-scope (TTS) and over-the-wire (OTW) techniques. In the TTS technique, the stent is advanced over the guide wire through the working channel of the endoscope and placed beyond the stricture. The stent is then deployed under endoscopic and fluoroscopic guidance (**Figs. 3 and 4**). When using the OTW technique, the endoscope is withdrawn leaving the guide wire in place. The stent is then advanced over the guide wire under fluoroscopic guidance. The endoscope can also be placed alongside the delivery catheter for endoscopic visualization of the proximal end of the stent to effect precise positioning.

SEMS are deployed starting at the distal end of the delivery catheter with the exception of one stent, namely the Boston Scientific Proximal Release Ultraflex stent. The delivery device of this stent incorporates a unique-knit outer sheath that unravels from the proximal end of the stent distally, allowing the stent to crown from the proximal end. Gentle back-tension is generally required because of the tendency for the stent to advance forward during deployment. Some stents can be reconstrained and adjusted during deployment until the radiopaque marker indicating the point of unreconstraint has been reached. The degree of stent foreshortening is variable among commercially available SEMS (**Figs. 5 and 6**), but must be taken into account

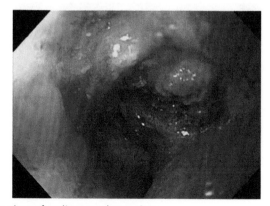

Fig. 1. Endoscopic view of malignant obstruction.

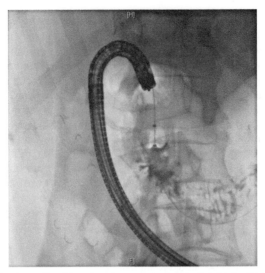

Fig. 2. Fluoroscopic view of guide-wire placement and contrast injection.

during stent positioning and deployment. The stent should be evaluated fluoroscopically once fully deployed to ensure each end of the stent is flared, producing a waist.

GASTRODUODENAL STENTS
Indication

Malignant gastroduodenal obstruction is associated with a poor quality of life, owing to limited oral intake and poor nutritional status. The most common causes of malignant upper gastrointestinal tract obstruction include cancers of the pancreas, stomach, ampulla of Vater, and bile duct, as well as metastatic disease. Patients often suffer from debilitating nausea, vomiting, malnutrition, weight loss, and dehydration. Traditional management has consisted of surgical gastrojejunostomy with combined hepaticojejunostomy in patients with concomitant biliary obstruction.[4,5] However, this surgical approach carries a high morbidity and mortality.[6,7] Gastroduodenal stents

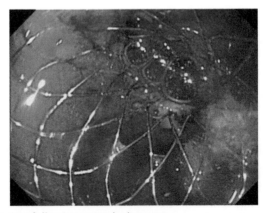

Fig. 3. Endoscopic view following stent deployment.

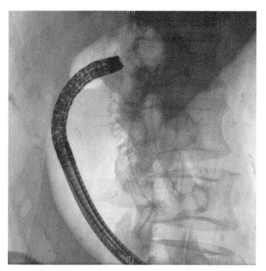

Fig. 4. Fluoroscopic view of deployed stent.

offer a nonsurgical alternative for palliation of obstructive symptoms to patients with a short life expectancy and poor prognosis.

Stent placement has been recommended in patients with limited life expectancy and poor quality of life, whereas surgery is generally reserved for patients with better overall health status and longer life expectancy. The most frequently used assessment tool to determine a patient's quality of life and performance status is the World Health Organization performance status (WHO status) (**Table 2**).

In a prospective study of 101 patients with malignant gastric outlet obstruction, patients with incomplete self-care (WHO status 3–4) had a significantly decreased 3-month survival rate of 26% compared with 60% for patients with complete self-care (WHO status 0–2). Additional poor prognostic indicators included patients with a high baseline pain score and use of pain medication stronger than morphine. Thirty-day survival rate was less than 10% in patients with all 3 prognostic indicators.[8]

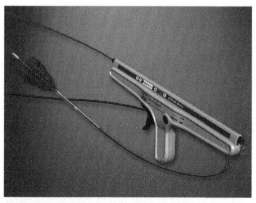

Fig. 5. Evolution colonic controlled-release stent. (Permission for use granted by Cook Medical Incorporated, Bloomington, Indiana.)

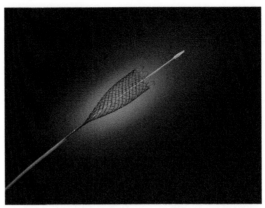

Fig. 6. Wallflex duodenal stent. (*Courtesy of* Boston Scientific, Natick, MA; with permission.)

Therefore, patients with a WHO performance status of 3 to 4 and other poor prognostic signs are the best candidates for endoscopic stent placement.

Outcomes

Several studies have reported on the efficacy of gastroduodenal stent placement for palliation of obstructive symptoms. In a systematic review of 44 studies, technical success defined by adequate positioning and deployment of the stent was successful in 972 of 1012 (96%) patients.[9] Relief of obstructive symptoms and/or improvement in oral intake defined as clinical success was achieved in 890 of 1000 (89%) patents.

Small, prospective controlled trials have been published within the past few years comparing gastroduodenal stent placement and palliative surgical bypass. In the largest multicenter prospective trial to date, Jeurnink and colleagues[10] randomized 18 patients to gastrojejunostomy and 21 to stent placement. Median time to tolerate at least soft solids was shorter following stent placement compared with gastrojejunostomy (median 5 days vs 8 days, $P<.01$). Hospital stay was also shorter in patients undergoing stent placement (median 7 days vs 15 days, $P = .04$). No major complications were observed in the surgical group, whereas 6 major complications occurred in 4 patients undergoing stent placement. When stent obstruction was excluded as a major complication, no differences in complication rates were found. There was no difference in median survival (stent 56 days vs surgery 78 days, $P = .19$). Longterm outcomes at 2 months favored patients who had undergone gastrojejunostomy as they were better able to tolerate food intake, had less recurrent obstructive symptoms, and had fewer reinterventions (10 in 7 stended patients vs 2 in 2 surgically treated patients, $P<.01$). Based on these results it has been suggested that stent placement is preferred in patients with a life expectancy shorter than 2 months. Initial

Table 2 World Health Organization performance status (WHO status)	
WHO 0	Fully active, able to carry on all predisease activities without restriction
WHO 1	Restricted in physically strenuous activity but able to carry out light work
WHO 2	Up and about more than 50% of waking hours
WHO 3	Confined to a bed or chair 50% or more of waking hours
WHO 4	Completely disabled; totally confined to bed or chair

procedure-related costs, as well as the cost of follow-up care, were compared in the same cohort of 39 patients.[11] Total overall costs were higher for surgically treated patients compared with stent placement (€12,433 vs €8819). This discrepancy was mainly due to higher initial costs of gastrojejunostomy related to a longer hospital stay. There was no difference in follow-up costs including the need for reintervention.

In a recent systematic review of 6 prospective studies comparing stent placement with surgical gastrojejunostomy, the findings of the aforementioned studies were confirmed, showing higher technical success, more rapid improvement of food intake, shorter hospital stay, and lower costs.[12] No difference was observed in clinical success, length of survival, and mortality. Because of the potential improved quality of life in patients with an overall limited life expectancy, faster relief of obstructive symptoms, and minimally invasive nature of endoluminal prosthetic deployment, endoscopic stent placement may be the preferred modality for palliation of obstructive symptoms in malignant gastroduodenal obstruction.

Complications

Severe complications from endoscopic gastroduodenal stent placement are rare. Data published from a systematic review of 606 patients showed a perforation rate of 0.7% and bleeding in 0.5%. Stent migration occurred in 5%.[13] These findings are similar to the results from an international prospective multicenter registry with reported complications of bleeding (3%), stent migration (1.5%), and perforation (0.5%).

One of the shortcomings of stent placement is stent occlusion as a result of tumor ingrowth or overgrowth, occurring in 12% to 17% of patients[13,14] Management of stent occlusion has usually consisted of placing a second stent within the occluded stent, termed the stent-in-stent, nested stent, or coaxial stenting technique, but available data on the success of this technique are limited.[15] In a retrospective Korean study of 77 patients with malignant gastric outlet obstruction, stent-in-stent placement was technically successful in all patients while obstructive symptoms improved in 68 of 77 (88%) patients.[16] Secondary stent malfunction occurred in 26 of 77 (34%) patients with a stent patency of 165 days. The most common cause of secondary stent malfunction was tumor ingrowth, occurring in 50% of patients. Both uncovered (66%) and covered (34%) stents were used in this study, and no differences were observed in secondary stent malfunction or secondary stent patency. Survival time of longer than 100 days and palliative chemotherapy were predictive of secondary stent malfunction.

Retrospective studies have suggested that chemotherapy is associated with improved stent patency.[17–19] The relationship between response to chemotherapy based on computed tomography imaging and stent-related outcomes was studied in 113 patients who underwent pyloric stent placement and palliative chemotherapy for gastric adenocarcinoma.[20] In this retrospective review, response to chemotherapy did not affect restenosis or stent migration. In addition, a long time to disease progression (>8 weeks) and first-line chemotherapy were protective factors against stent occlusion.

COLONIC STENTS
Indication

Acute colonic obstruction is a common presentation of colorectal cancer, occurring in 10% to 30% of new cases presenting in the left colon.[21–23] Emergency surgical decompression has traditionally been performed in this setting, because of the potential progression to bowel ischemia and perforation if left untreated. While general consensus supports resection and primary anastomosis for acute right-sided colonic obstruction, management of left-sided obstruction is more controversial.[24] Emergency surgery typically requires a 2-stage procedure, with initial surgical resection and creation of an ostomy followed by reanastomosis at a later date. Emergent surgery is also associated with morbidity approaching 40%.[25,26] Furthermore, future colostomy reversal is not done following emergency surgery in up to 40% of patients, owing to rapidly progressive disease or medical comorbidities.[27–29] Primary anastomosis is generally avoided in acute left-sided colonic obstruction because of the high risk of anastomotic leak.[30] Alternatively, colonic stent placement may be performed to relieve acute obstruction and serve as a bridge to surgery. This approach allows for effective bowel preparation and eventual surgical resection with primary anastomosis in a 1-stage operation.[31]

Metastatic colorectal cancer is discovered at the time of diagnosis in up to 20% of patients.[32] In patients with metastatic disease or who are not otherwise candidates for surgical curative resection, colorectal stent placement may be performed for definitive palliation of obstructive symptoms.

Outcomes

The efficacy of colorectal stent placement has been rigorously studied. In a systematic review of 88 studies, colorectal stent placement was technically successful at a median rate of 96% (range 66%–100%) and clinically successful at a median rate of 92% (range 46%–100%).[33] Successful stent placement was achieved in these studies regardless of the indication for stent placement or the cause of the obstruction.

Bridge to Surgery

Four randomized controlled trials have been conducted to evaluate colorectal stents as a bridge to surgery compared with emergency surgery in acute malignant left-sided large bowel obstruction.[34–37] A meta-analysis of these 4 studies including 234 patients was performed, with 116 patients in the stent group and 118 in the emergency surgery group.[38] Overall technical success in patients undergoing stent placement was achieved in 82 of 116 (71%) patients, and clinical success was demonstrated in 80 of 116 (69%) patients. This outcome compares with a systematic review by Sebastian and colleagues,[39] which reported a technical and clinical success rate of 92% and 72%, respectively, and a Cochrane review indicating 86% technical and 78% clinical success.[40] The meta-analysis data were also significant for stent placement associated with significantly higher successful primary anastomosis and lower overall stoma rates. No significant differences were observed in permanent stoma creation, in-hospital mortality, anastomotic leak, and 30-day reoperation rates.

Three out of the 4 clinical trials included in the meta-analysis were discontinued prematurely. In the study by Alcantara and colleagues,[34] the rate of anastomotic leak in the emergency surgery group was significantly higher than in patients who had received a stent as a bridge to surgery. Pirlet and colleagues[36] noted a 54% technical failure of stent placement, and the trial had to be stopped owing to 3 colonic perforations during stent placement. Interim analysis by Van Hooft and colleagues[37] revealed an increased absolute risk of 30-day morbidity in patients who had received colorectal stents. Because of these conflicting results, it has been suggested that preoperative colonic stent placement may best be reserved for patients with high preoperative morbidity and mortality, in institutions with technical expertise in enteral stent placement.[41]

Palliation

Palliative colonic stent placement offers relief of obstructive symptoms and potentially improved quality of life in patients with advanced disease. In a recent retrospective review of 88 patients over an 8-year period, compared with palliative surgery colonic stent placement was associated with a shorter hospital stay (7.2 vs 12.3 days, $P = .001$), lower stoma formation (16.7% vs 38.5%, $P = .021$), and shorter interval to initiation of chemotherapy. (8.1 vs 21.7 days, $P = .001$).[42] An Italian multicenter experience showed that 75% of patients who underwent colonic stent placement for palliation were able to avoid a colostomy.[43]

Lee and colleagues[44] reported on the long-term efficacy of palliative stent placement compared with surgical palliation in a retrospective study of 144 patients. In this study, the median patency of SEMS was comparable with that of surgery (229 vs 268 days, $P = .239$), when taking into account reinterventions for endoscopically managed stent complications. In a retrospective review of the Mayo Clinic experience, long-term (6-month) clinical success rate of palliative stent placement was 77.2% with a mean stent patency of 145 days.[45] Taken together, these studies reflect the safety and efficacy of palliative stent placement in comparison with palliative surgery.

A Dutch multicenter, randomized controlled trial was designed to evaluate the effectiveness of endoscopic stent placement compared with surgery in patients with stage IV left-sided colorectal cancer.[46] Unfortunately, the study had to be terminated owing to an unusually high rate of stent-related perforations after enrollment of 21 patients. Six out of 11 patients in the stent group experienced delayed perforation, resulting in 3 deaths. Possible explanations for the unexpected high complication rate may be related to administration of chemotherapy and the design of the particular stent used in this study.

Complications

A long-term retrospective study of patients undergoing colorectal stent placement as a bridge to surgery or for palliative purposes at the Mayo Clinic revealed an overall stent complication rate of 24%.[45] The most common adverse events included stent occlusion (7.7%), perforation (7.7%), and stent migration (6.9%). Minor complications such as bleeding, infection, and tenesmus occurred in 0.9%, 3%, and 2.1%, respectively.

The most feared complication following colonic stent placement is procedural or delayed perforation. This issue has gained an increasing amount of attention, especially after the premature closure of the aforementioned prospective multicenter Dutch trial. In a review of 82 articles including 2287 patients, an overall perforation rate of 4.9% was found.[47] No significant difference in perforation rates was discovered between bridge to surgery and palliative indications. Risk factors for perforation included chemotherapy, steroids, and radiation therapy. Additional predictors of procedure and stent-related complications include complete bowel obstruction, endoscopist experience, stent diameter, and pre–stent-deployment dilation.[45]

Bevacizumab has increasingly been associated with colonic perforation, and in one study nearly tripled the risk of perforation.[45] Manes and colleagues[43] conducted a multicenter retrospective analysis over a 3-year period and found that bevacizumab was associated with a 19.6-fold increase in the risk of perforation. Of interest, the perforation risk may actually be independent of stent placement. In a meta-analysis of 17 randomized controlled trials, bevacizumab was found to increase significantly the risk of gastrointestinal perforation in comparison with controls.[48] It is hypothesized that the antiangiogenic drug effect may damage the structure and function of gastrointestinal vasculature, resulting in ischemic perforation.[49]

SUMMARY

Colorectal stent placement offers a minimally invasive approach for relief of malignant bowel obstruction. Stent placement is safe and effective in carefully selected patients as a bridge to surgery or for definitive palliation of obstruction. Concerns remain regarding the long-term efficacy of stent placement and related complications. Future studies are needed to identify patients who are the best candidates for stent placement.

REFERENCES

1. Dohmoto M, Rupp KD, Hohlbach G. Endoscopically-implanted prosthesis in rectal carcinoma. Dtsch Med Wochenschr 1990;115:915 [in German].
2. Spinelli P, Dal Fante M, Mancini A. Self-expanding mesh stent for endoscopic palliation of rectal obstructing tumors: a preliminary report. Surg Endosc 1992; 6:72–4.
3. Duerig TP, Pelton A, Stockel D. An overview of nitinol medical applications. Mater Sci Eng A-structural Materials Properties Microst 1999;275:149–60.
4. Lillemoe KD, Pitt HA. Palliation. Surgical and otherwise. Cancer 1996;78:605–14.
5. Sohn TA, Lillemoe KD, Cameron JL, et al. Surgical palliation of unresectable peri-ampullary adenocarcinoma in the 1990s. J Am Coll Surg 1999;188:658–66 [discussion: 66–9].
6. Bozzetti F, Bonfanti G, Audisio RA, et al. Prognosis of patients after palliative surgical procedures for carcinoma of the stomach. Surg Gynecol Obstet 1987; 164:151–4.
7. Weaver DW, Wiencek RG, Bouwman DL, et al. Gastrojejunostomy: is it helpful for patients with pancreatic cancer? Surgery 1987;102:608–13.
8. van Hooft JE, Dijkgraaf MG, Timmer R, et al. Independent predictors of survival in patients with incurable malignant gastric outlet obstruction: a multicenter prospective observational study. Scand J Gastroenterol 2010;45:1217–22.
9. Jeurnink SM, van Eijck CH, Steyerberg EW, et al. Stent versus gastrojejunostomy for the palliation of gastric outlet obstruction: a systematic review. BMC Gastro-enterol 2007;7:18.
10. Jeurnink SM, Steyerberg EW, van Hooft JE, et al. Surgical gastrojejunostomy or endoscopic stent placement for the palliation of malignant gastric outlet obstruc-tion (SUSTENT study): a multicenter randomized trial. Gastrointest Endosc 2010; 71:490–9.
11. Jeurnink SM, Polinder S, Steyerberg EW, et al. Cost comparison of gastrojejunos-tomy versus duodenal stent placement for malignant gastric outlet obstruction. J Gastroenterol 2010;45:537–43.
12. Zheng B, Wang X, Ma B, et al. Endoscopic stenting versus gastrojejunostomy for palliation of malignant gastric outlet obstruction. Dig Endosc 2012;24:71–8.
13. Dormann A, Meisner S, Verin N, et al. Self-expanding metal stents for gastrodu-odenal malignancies: systematic review of their clinical effectiveness. Endoscopy 2004;36:543–50.
14. Costamagna G, Tringali A, Spicak J, et al. Treatment of malignant gastroduodenal obstruction with a nitinol self-expanding metal stent: an international prospective multicentre registry. Dig Liver Dis 2012;44:37–43.
15. Homs MY, Steyerberg EW, Kuipers EJ, et al. Causes and treatment of recurrent dysphagia after self-expanding metal stent placement for palliation of esopha-geal carcinoma. Endoscopy 2004;36:880–6.

16. Park JC, Park JJ, Cheoi K, et al. Clinical outcomes of secondary stent-in-stent self-expanding metal stent placement for primary stent malfunction in malignant gastric outlet obstruction. Dig Liver Dis 2012;44(12):999–1005.

17. Kim JH, Song HY, Shin JH, et al. Metallic stent placement in the palliative treatment of malignant gastroduodenal obstructions: prospective evaluation of results and factors influencing outcome in 213 patients. Gastrointest Endosc 2007;66: 256–64.

18. Telford JJ, Carr-Locke DL, Baron TH, et al. Palliation of patients with malignant gastric outlet obstruction with the enteral Wallstent: outcomes from a multicenter study. Gastrointest Endosc 2004;60:916–20.

19. Cho YK, Kim SW, Hur WH, et al. Clinical outcomes of self-expandable metal stent and prognostic factors for stent patency in gastric outlet obstruction caused by gastric cancer. Dig Dis Sci 2010;55:668–74.

20. Kim CG, Park SR, Choi IJ, et al. Effect of chemotherapy on the outcome of self-expandable metallic stents in gastric cancer patients with malignant outlet obstruction. Endoscopy 2012;44:807–12.

21. Deans GT, Krukowski ZH, Irwin ST. Malignant obstruction of the left colon. Br J Surg 1994;81:1270–6.

22. Rault A, Collet D, Sa Cunha A, et al. Surgical management of obstructed colonic cancer. Ann Chir 2005;130:331–5 [in French].

23. Tekkis PP, Kinsman R, Thompson MR, et al. The Association of Coloproctology of Great Britain and Ireland study of large bowel obstruction caused by colorectal cancer. Ann Surg 2004;240:76–81.

24. Finan PJ, Campbell S, Verma R, et al. The management of malignant large bowel obstruction: ACPGBI position statement. Colorectal Dis 2007;9(Suppl 4): 1–17.

25. Sjo OH, Larsen S, Lunde OC, et al. Short term outcome after emergency and elective surgery for colon cancer. Colorectal Dis 2009;11:733–9.

26. Villar JM, Martinez AP, Villegas MT, et al. Surgical options for malignant left-sided colonic obstruction. Surg Today 2005;35:275–81.

27. Pearce NW, Scott SD, Karran SJ. Timing and method of reversal of Hartmann's procedure. Br J Surg 1992;79:839–41.

28. Desai DC, Brennan EJ Jr, Reilly JF, et al. The utility of the Hartmann procedure. Am J Surg 1998;175:152–4.

29. Koruth NM, Krukowski ZH, Youngson GG, et al. Intra-operative colonic irrigation in the management of left-sided large bowel emergencies. Br J Surg 1985;72: 708–11.

30. Kingham TP, Pachter HL. Colonic anastomotic leak: risk factors, diagnosis, and treatment. J Am Coll Surg 2009;208:269–78.

31. Park IJ, Choi GS, Kang BM, et al. Comparison of one-stage managements of obstructing left-sided colon and rectal cancer: stent-laparoscopic approach vs. intraoperative colonic lavage. J Gastrointest Surg 2009;13:960–5.

32. Fast stats: an interactive tool for access to SEER cancer statistics. Surveillance Research Program, National Cancer Institute. Available at: http://seer.cancer. gov/faststats. Accessed August 28, 2012.

33. Watt AM, Faragher IG, Griffin TT, et al. Self-expanding metallic stents for relieving malignant colorectal obstruction: a systematic review. Ann Surg 2007; 246:24–30.

34. Alcantara M, Serra-Aracil X, Falco J, et al. Prospective, controlled, randomized study of intraoperative colonic lavage versus stent placement in obstructive left-sided colonic cancer. World J Surg 2011;35:1904–10.

35. Cheung HY, Chung CC, Tsang WW, et al. Endolaparoscopic approach vs conventional open surgery in the treatment of obstructing left-sided colon cancer: a randomized controlled trial. Arch Surg 2009;144:1127–32.
36. Pirlet IA, Slim K, Kwiatkowski F, et al. Emergency preoperative stenting versus surgery for acute left-sided malignant colonic obstruction: a multicenter randomized controlled trial. Surg Endosc 2011;25:1814–21.
37. van Hooft JE, Bemelman WA, Oldenburg B, et al. Colonic stenting versus emergency surgery for acute left-sided malignant colonic obstruction: a multicentre randomised trial. Lancet Oncol 2011;12:344–52.
38. Tan CJ, Dasari BV, Gardiner K. Systematic review and meta-analysis of randomized clinical trials of self-expanding metallic stents as a bridge to surgery versus emergency surgery for malignant left-sided large bowel obstruction. Br J Surg 2012;99:469–76.
39. Sebastian S, Johnston S, Geoghegan T, et al. Pooled analysis of the efficacy and safety of self-expanding metal stenting in malignant colorectal obstruction. Am J Gastroenterol 2004;99:2051–7.
40. Sagar J. Colorectal stents for the management of malignant colonic obstructions. Cochrane Database Syst Rev 2011;(11):CD007378.
41. Song LM, Baron TH. Stenting for acute malignant colonic obstruction: a bridge to nowhere? Lancet Oncol 2011;12:314–5.
42. Lee WS, Baek JH, Kang JM, et al. The outcome after stent placement or surgery as the initial treatment for obstructive primary tumor in patients with stage IV colon cancer. Am J Surg 2012;203:715–9.
43. Manes G, de Bellis M, Fuccio L, et al. Endoscopic palliation in patients with incurable malignant colorectal obstruction by means of self-expanding metal stent: analysis of results and predictors of outcomes in a large multicenter series. Arch Surg 2011;146:1157–62.
44. Lee HJ, Hong SP, Cheon JH, et al. Long-term outcome of palliative therapy for malignant colorectal obstruction in patients with unresectable metastatic colorectal cancers: endoscopic stenting versus surgery. Gastrointest Endosc 2011; 73:535–42.
45. Small AJ, Coelho-Prabhu N, Baron TH. Endoscopic placement of self-expandable metal stents for malignant colonic obstruction: long-term outcomes and complication factors. Gastrointest Endosc 2010;71:560–72.
46. van Hooft JE, Fockens P, Marinelli AW, et al. Early closure of a multicenter randomized clinical trial of endoscopic stenting versus surgery for stage IV left-sided colorectal cancer. Endoscopy 2008;40:184–91.
47. Datye A, Hersh J. Colonic perforation after stent placement for malignant colorectal obstruction–causes and contributing factors. Minim Invasive Ther Allied Technol 2011;20:133–40.
48. Cennamo V, Fuccio L, Mutri V, et al. Does stent placement for advanced colon cancer increase the risk of perforation during bevacizumab-based therapy? Clin Gastroenterol Hepatol 2009;7:1174–6.
49. Hapani S, Chu D, Wu S. Risk of gastrointestinal perforation in patients with cancer treated with bevacizumab: a meta-analysis. Lancet Oncol 2009;10:559–68.

Endoscopy in the Management of Obesity

Shelby Sullivan, MD

KEYWORDS

- Weight regain • Endoscopic bariatric revision • Endoscopic bariatric therapy
- Intragastric balloon • Duodenal jejunal bypass liner

KEY POINTS

- Obesity affects more than one third of adults in the United States and is associated with increased morbidity, mortality, and health care costs.
- Current treatment options include medical management with therapeutic lifestyle change and pharmacotherapy, as well as bariatric surgery; however, these treatments have limitations.
- Endoscopic therapies are emerging as potential tools to address the limitations of the current obesity therapies.

The latest National Health and Nutrition Examination Survey data from 2009 through 2010 indicates 35.5% of adult men and 35.8% of adult women in the United States have a body mass index (BMI) of >30 kg/m^2.[1] Obesity adversely affects every organ system, and it increases morbidity and mortality.[2–4] In addition, recent data suggests that there is a 2- to 3-fold increase for incremental health care costs in obese adults in the United States compared with normal weight adults.[5] Given the prevalence of obesity and its associated morbidity, mortality, and increasing health care costs, it is imperative that the medical community addresses this disease.

Unfortunately, current treatment options for obesity are limited. Therapeutic lifestyle change (TLC) consisting of diet, exercise, and behavior modification results in up to 10% short-term weight loss, but 5% or less weight loss in the long term.[6] Weight loss medications increase weight loss by 3% to 5% over placebo and are more likely to result in 10% weight loss in patients than TLC alone[7]; however, medical therapy must be continued long term to maintain any weight loss achieved with the medication. Bariatric surgery has been shown to be superior to TLC[8,9] and pharmacotherapy[10] for weight loss and weight maintenance, and remains the most effective

Disclosures: Site investigator for both ReShape Duo (ReShape Medical) and EndoBarrier (GI Dynamics).
Division of Gastroenterology, Center for Human Nutrition, Washington University School of Medicine, 660 South Euclid Avenue, Campus Box 8124, St Louis, MO 63110, USA
E-mail address: ssulliva@dom.wustl.edu

Gastrointest Endoscopy Clin N Am 23 (2013) 165–175
http://dx.doi.org/10.1016/j.giec.2012.10.009
1052-5157/13/$ – see front matter Published by Elsevier Inc.

treatment option available for obesity. Although short-term costs for the surgery and postoperative complications are high, long-term cost–benefit analyses favor bariatric surgery over medical management of obesity.[11] Minor postoperative complications occur frequently, but serious complications occur in 5% or fewer of post bariatric surgery patients and the mortality rate is low.[12] However, 2 issues continue to plague bariatric surgery: Failure of weight loss or weight regain and limited access to surgery. Although the number of bariatric procedures performed per year has increased from 9189 in 1993 to 124,838 in 2008,[13] this only represents approximately 1% of obese persons who qualify for a bariatric surgical procedure.[12] Endoscopic bariatric procedures have emerged as potential options that not only address both of these issues, but also have reduced associated morbidity and mortality as well.

ENDOSCOPIC THERAPY FOR WEIGHT LOSS FAILURE

Weight regain has been reported in long-term studies, capturing patient weight 10 years or more after the original bariatric surgical procedure.[14–16] In the Swedish Obesity Study, 8.8% of Roux-en-Y gastric bypass (RYGB) patients and 25% of adjustable gastric banding patients maintained less than 5% of their weight loss at 10 years.[14] Similar rates of weight loss failure at 10 or more years of follow-up, as defined by end BMI compared with starting BMI,[17] were seen in patients after RYGB and Biliopancreatic Diversion (BPD), but were higher in patients with higher preoperative BMI.[15,16,18]

Although multiple factors likely play a role in weight regain, the factors that may be treated by endoscopists include gastro-gastric fistulas, stoma dilation, and pouch dilation. Some controversy exists regarding the role of stoma and pouch dilation in weight regain. Multiple early studies did not show a correlation between pouch diameter and weight loss[19–24]; however, some early studies did show a correlation,[25] even in the setting of extensive behavior modification therapy.[26] More recently, both pouch size[27] and stoma diameter have been shown to be significantly correlated with weight loss failure or weight regain in both univariate and multivariate analyses,[28,29] but not in all studies.[30] Heneghan and colleagues[29] found small, but significant differences pouch length (5.0 ± 2.4 vs 5.8 ± 2.6 cm; $P = .005$) and stoma diameter (2.1 ± 0.8 vs 2.5 ± 1.0 cm; $P<.001$) in the control (no weight regain) compared with weight regain groups, respectively. Failure to lose weight or weight regain has been treated by bariatric surgical revision with mixed outcomes. Weight loss has been demonstrated, but the surgical complication rates are higher than with the index procedure.[31–34] Given the risk of revisional surgery, endoscopic approaches including the use of sclerosants to decrease stoma diameter, as well as decreasing stoma and pouch size with suturing, tissue plication, or clips have been investigated as safer options compared with surgery.

Sclerotherapy of dilated gastrojejunostomies was first described in 2003,[35] and since then a number of series using sclerotherapy for dilated stomas have been published with weight loss or weight stabilization in 50% to 91.6% of patients at 1 year.[36–40] The largest of these series included 231 patients with weight regain and an average baseline gastrojejunostomy stoma diameter that was 19 mm. These patients were treated with an average of 2 sclerotherapy sessions and 16 mL of sodium morrhuate injected at each session.[40] The average weight loss 6 months after sclerotherapy was 18% of the weight that had been regained, and 76% of patients lost more weight or maintained their 6-month weight loss at 12 months. Complications included bleeding (2.4% immediate and 0.2% delayed), abdominal pain requiring admission (0.5%), and small ulcers on repeat endoscopy (1%). Baseline stoma diameter was not a predictor of response to sclerotherapy.

The Endocinch Suturing System (C.R. BARD Inc, Murray Hill, NJ, USA) was piloted by Thompson and colleagues[41] in 2006. The authors used a technique of mucosal ablation with argon plasma coagulation followed by placement of 2 sutures on average and then tightening the sutures to form tissue plications. The average stoma diameter was reduced to 10 mm (68% reduction), and patients had an average excess weight loss of 23.4%. This device has also been studied in a randomized, double-blinded, sham-controlled, multicenter trial of 77 patients. Patients included in the study had baseline stoma diameters of more than 20 mm. The authors achieved a gastrojejunostomy of 10 mm or less in 89% of patients randomized to the treatment arm with an average number of 4 sutures placed. A trend was seen in the intention-to-treat analysis with more weight loss in the treatment group compared with the control group ($4.2 \pm 5.4\%$ and $1.9 \pm 5.2\%$; $P = .066$) at 6 months.[42]

The Incisionless Operating Platform (USGI Medical, San Clemente, CA, USA) is a tissue plication system that places expandable tissue anchors to hold tissue together. Two small pilot studies of decreasing stoma diameter and pouch length in patients with weight regain after RYGB demonstrated short-term weight loss of 7.8 to 8.8 kg at 3 months.[43,44] Data from a multicenter registry of 116 patients reported 32% (6.5 ± 6.5 kg) of the regained weight was lost at 6 months with stoma diameter reduced by 50% to 11.5 mm, and pouch length reduced by 44% to 3.3 cm.[45] At 12 months post-procedure, 73 of 112 subjects with successful procedures had a total weight loss of 5.9 ± 1.1 kg.[46]

The StomaphyX device (EndoGastric Solutions Inc, Redmond, WA, USA) is a tissue plication device that uses polypropylene H-fasteners to approximate serosal surfaces. This device was first used to treat weight regain with 39 patients who were at least 2 years out from RYGB and had gained at least 10% of their lowest weight.[47] Excess body weight loss was 19.5% 12 months post-procedure; however, only 6 of 39 patients returned for the 12-month follow-up. Another study of 64 patients used an average of 23 H-fasteners and reported a 33% decrease in gastric pouch length and the stoma was reduced from 22 to 9 mm.[48] The average weight loss was 7.3 kg, but the mean follow-up was only 5.8 months. Two other small studies have shown weight loss after endoscopic revision with StomaphyX.[49,50]

Over-The-Scope-Clips (Ovesco, Tubingen, Germany) have also been used to reduce stoma diameter to treat weight regain after bariatric surgery. One study reported 94 subjects whose stoma diameter was reduced from 35 to 8 mm with placement of up to 2 Over-The-Scope-Clips placed on opposite sides of the stoma.[51] Mean BMI decreased from 32.8 ± 1.9 to 27.4 ± 3.8 kg/m^2 at 12 months; however, 2 patients requiring dilation of the stoma to 12 mm owing to persistent dysphagia.

Although these case series are encouraging, further research in endoscopic therapy of weight regain after bariatric surgery is needed. First, only one endoscopic bariatric revision procedure has been studied in a randomized, double-blind, sham-controlled study, and only a trend was seen toward more weight loss in the treatment group.[42] This may in part be due to either patient selection or the underlying cause for the stoma and pouch dilation, which has yet to be determined. Based on the variability in the pre-endoscopic revision stoma and pouch diameter seen in these cases series as well as the study by Heneghan and colleagues demonstrating statistically different but clinically similar stoma diameter between patients with weight regain and those maintaining their weight loss, it is unclear which patients are most likely to benefit from these procedures. However, given the weight loss seen in many patients and the significantly decreased risks associated with endoscopic stoma and pouch revision compared with surgical revision, endoscopic treatment of weight regain after bariatric surgery remains a promising therapeutic option.

PRIMARY ENDOSCOPIC BARIATRIC THERAPY

Endoscopic bariatric therapy (EBT) is still in its infancy, and currently no EBT devices have been approved for use in the United States; however, there are many advantages to EBT compared with traditional bariatric surgery. First, although weight loss with EBT is likely to be less than most bariatric surgical procedures, EBT is associated with lower complication rates and shorter recovery times than bariatric surgery. Both the lower risk profile and decreased recovery time may increase the number of patients willing to undergo a weight loss procedure. In addition, because most EBT only require conscious sedation, sicker patients who may not be good candidates for surgery may still qualify for endoscopic placement of a device. Further, although bariatric surgery is the most effective therapy for weight loss at the patient level, it is limited by the number of patients who can be treated per year, restricting its effect on obesity treatment at the population level. Owing to both the number of practicing gastroenterologists and the short amount of time required for these procedures compared with bariatric operative procedures, the number of patients who could undergo EBT potentially dwarfs the number of patients who are able to undergo bariatric surgery per year, making more of an impact on obesity at the population level. Multiple devices have been or are currently in the development and testing stages for EBT; however, for the purposes of this review, only technologies that have published data and are still viable are discussed.

INTRAGASTRIC BALLOON

The intragastric balloon (IGB) is a device that was designed to occupy space and cause gastric distension with the goal of decreasing food intake. The first IGB device, the Garren-Edwards Gastric Bubble, was approved for use by the US Food and Drug Administration in 1985; however, it was taken off of the market in 1992 owing to both complications (including damage to the gastric mucosa and balloon deflation with subsequent small bowel obstruction) and lack of difference between the device and TLC in sham-controlled trials.[52–59] These 2 issues were thought to be related to the design of the device itself. First, the device volume was only 220 mL when distended, and evidence suggests that a volume of at least 400 mL is needed for a reduction of food intake,[60] and the device had a cylindrical shape with edges, which damaged the mucosa. In addition, it was made from polyurethane that was too easily deflated. Several new designs including the BioEnterics IGB (BIB; Allergan, Irvine, CA, USA), ReShape Duo (ReShape Medical, San Clemente, CA, USA; **Fig. 1**.), the Heliosphere IGB (Helioscopie, Vienne, France), and the Spatz Adjustable Balloon System (Spatz FGIA, Jericho, NY, USA) have been developed and address the issues surrounding the failure of the Garren-Edwards gastric bubble. Although these devices have different designs to decrease balloon rupture and migration, they all have eliminated edges to reduce mucosal damage and have increased device volume to induce an effect on food intake.

Data suggest the current IGBs are effective at inducing weight loss significantly greater than lifestyle therapy alone or pharmacotherapy. A randomized, controlled, cross-over trial demonstrated superiority of IGBs to pharmacotherapy with sibuatramine ($14.5 \pm 1.2\%$ compared with $9.1 \pm 1.5\%$ total body weight loss; $P<.05$).[61] Imaz and colleagues[62] performed a meta-analysis on 15 studies with a total of 3608 subjects receiving the BIB. Mean weight loss across studies was 14.7 kg or 12.2% of total body weight. Only 2 randomized controlled trials were included; however, these 2 studies attributed 6.7-kg of the weight loss to the BIB. Complications were rare, but included 26 cases of obstruction in the gastrointestinal tract, 4 cases of

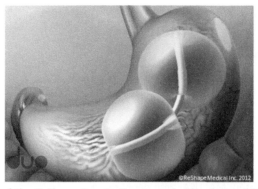

Fig. 1. Illustration of the ReShape Duo in the stomach after being filled with 450 mL of saline in each of the balloons. (*Courtesy of* ReShape Medical, Inc, San Clemente, CA, USA; with permission.)

gastric perforation, and 2 deaths related to gastric perforations. Four percent of subjects underwent early removal of the BIB. These studies did not have long follow-up; however, a subsequent study of 195 subjects who completed 60 months of follow-up demonstrated a 13% excess weight loss with 23% of subjects maintaining more than 20% excess weight loss.[63] In addition, IGBs have been evaluated for short-term weight loss before surgeries such as laparoscopic gastric bypass with a significant decrease in weight compared with control subjects and a 75% reduction in the composite endpoint of conversion to open gastric bypass, intensive care stay of longer than 2 days, or hospital stay of longer than 2 weeks ($P = .031$).[64]

Studies have also investigated the repeated use of IGB for long-term weight loss therapy. Genco and colleagues[65] reported 100 obese patients who were randomized to receive the IGB for 6 months followed by lifestyle therapy alone or IGB followed by another IGB placement 1 month later for 6 months. At 6 months, the percent excess weight loss was the same in the 2 groups ($43.5 \pm 21.1\%$ and $45.2 \pm 22.5\%$, respectively); however, at 13 months the percent excess weight loss was greater in patients receiving 2 consecutive IGB placements compared with the patients receiving 1 IGB placement followed by lifestyle therapy ($51.9 \pm 24.6\%$ and $25.1 \pm 26.2\%$, respectively). Another study with 5-year follow-up compared patients who requested repeated IGB compared with patients who had only 1 IGB placement and found no difference in percent of subjects with at least 10% total body weight loss at 5 years.[66]

Taken together, these data suggest that the current generation of IGBs have lower complication rates than the first generation of IGB. IGB placement is an effective tool for short-term weight loss, and preoperative weight loss with IGB may decrease complications in surgeries, such as bariatric surgery. Furthermore, some patients may be able to maintain a portion of the weight loss achieved with the IGB without further intervention, whereas some patients may benefit from further IGB placement. Additional research is needed to address these long-term management questions.

DUODENAL JEJUNAL BYPASS LINER

The duodenal jejunal bypass liner (DJBL; EndoBarrier, GI Dynamics, Boston, MA, USA; **Fig. 2**) is an endoscopically placed and retrieved impermeable liner that anchors in the duodenal bulb and extends 60 cm into the small bowel. The device is meant to mimic the effects of bypassing the duodenum in bariatric surgery. Although human

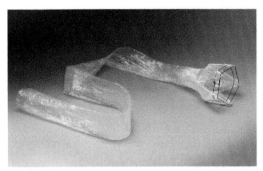

Fig. 2. Photograph of the EndoBarrier, a duodenal jejunal bypass liner. (*Courtesy of* GI Dynamics, Inc, Lexington, MA, USA; with permission.)

data examining the effects of bariatric surgery on glucose metabolism and multi-organ insulin sensitivity independent of weight loss are limited, recent data from animal models suggest that jejunal nutrient sensing after duodenal exclusion plays a role in the early improvement in glycemic control after duodenal jejunal bypass surgery.[67]

The first human experience with the DJBL was published in 2008 with 12 subjects in a 12-week, open-label, prospective study.[68] Although 2 subjects underwent explant at 9 days (owing to the position of the device placement), no serious adverse events occurred. Subjects lost 23.6% excess weight loss at 12 weeks and reportedly 4 subjects who had type 2 diabetes before device placement attained normal fasting serum glucose concentrations off of oral hypoglycemic medications, although the serum glucose concentrations were not reported. Since then, a few studies have been published for preoperative weight loss in patients who are candidates for bariatric surgery. A single-center, 12-week, randomized, controlled trial demonstrated a 22.1 ± 8% (n = 20) compared with 5.3% ± 6.6% (n = 4) excess weight loss in the DJBL compared with control groups (*P* = .02),[69] and a 12-week, multicenter, randomized, controlled trial with extension to 24 weeks in 3 subjects in the DJBL group, revealed a similar weight loss of 19.0 ± 10.9% compared with 6.9 ± 6.1% excess weight loss in the DJBL (n = 24) and control groups (n = 11; *P*<.002). A sham-controlled trial for preoperative weight loss, however, demonstrated 11.9 ± 1.4% compared with 2.7 ± 2% excess weight loss in the DJBL (n = 13) and control groups (n = 24), respectively (*P*<.05).[70] A 24-week, randomized, sham-controlled trial also demonstrated superiority of the DJBL over sham control for decreasing HbA1c in patients with type 2 diabetes (–2.4 ± 0.7% and –0.8 ± 0.4% in the DJBL and control groups respectively; *P*<.05).[71] In addition, an open-labeled study revealed a decrease in HbA1c (–2.3 ± 0.3%) in 13 subjects who completed 52 weeks of treatment with the DJBL.[72] It is important to note that 17% to 40% of subjects enrolled in these studies had early device removal predominantly due to gastrointestinal bleeding, abdominal pain, nausea and vomiting, anchor migration, or obstruction. However, few serious adverse events have been reported and no surgical interventions or deaths have been reported in relation to the DJBL.

TRANSORAL GASTRIC VOLUME REDUCTION

Transoral gastric volume reduction (**Fig. 3**) uses endoluminal suturing devices to reduce gastric volume to limit food intake; to date, 1 pilot study—the TRIM trial—has been reported.[73] The TRIM trial was an open-label, prospective, multicenter, single-arm feasibility study using the RESTORe Suturing System (Bard/Davol,

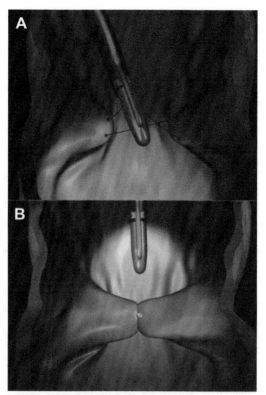

Fig. 3. *Panel A* Illustration of sutures being tightened with the RESTORe Suturing System. *Panel B* Illustration of a completed plication approximating the anterior and posterior walls of the stomach. (*From* Brethauer SA, Chand B, Schauer PR, et al. Transoral gastric volume reduction as intervention for weight management: 12-month follow-up of TRIM trial. Surg Obes Relat Dis 2012;8(3):296–303; with permission.)

Warwick, RI, USA) to plicate the anterior and posterior walls of the stomach, resulting in reduced gastric volume owing to the approximation of the anterior and posterior gastric walls. A total of 18 patients received an average of 6 plications; however, only 14 subjects completed 12 months of follow-up demonstrating a weight change of −11.0 ± 10.0 kg and 27.7 ± 21.9% excess weight loss. No serious adverse events occurred, but plication was only successful in 16 patients and at 12-month endoscopy all sutures had spontaneously released in 5 subjects.

SUMMARY

Endoscopic therapies for both primary treatment of obesity and weight regain after bariatric surgery have made significant advances. Although further research is necessary, these emerging technologies are poised to provide much needed additional tools for the management of obesity. This will allow endoscopists to fill an important void in the current spectrum of obesity therapy.

REFERENCES

1. Flegal KM, Carroll MD, Kit BK, et al. Prevalence of obesity and trends in the distribution of body mass index among US adults, 1999-2010. JAMA 2012;307:491–7.

2. Flegal KM, Graubard BI, Williamson DF, et al. Cause-specific excess deaths associated with underweight, overweight, and obesity. JAMA 2007;298:2028–37.
3. Katzmarzyk PT, Reeder BA, Elliott S, et al. Body mass index and risk of cardiovascular disease, cancer and all-cause mortality. Can J Public Health 2012;103: 147–51.
4. Peeters A, Barendregt JJ, Willekens F, et al. Obesity in adulthood and its consequences for life expectancy: a life-table analysis. Ann Intern Med 2003;138: 24–32.
5. Moriarty JP, Branda ME, Olsen KD, et al. The effects of incremental costs of smoking and obesity on health care costs among adults: a 7-year longitudinal study. J Occup Environ Med 2012;54:286–91.
6. Wadden TA, Butryn ML, Wilson C. Lifestyle modification for the management of obesity. Gastroenterology 2007;132:2226–38.
7. Rucker D, Padwal R, Li SK, et al. Long term pharmacotherapy for obesity and overweight: updated meta-analysis. BMJ 2007;335:1194–9.
8. Schauer PR, Kashyap SR, Wolski K, et al. Bariatric surgery versus intensive medical therapy in obese patients with diabetes. N Engl J Med 2012;366: 1567–76.
9. O'Brien PE, Dixon JB, Laurie C, et al. Treatment of mild to moderate obesity with laparoscopic adjustable gastric banding or an intensive medical program: a randomized trial. Ann Intern Med 2006;144:625–33.
10. Fabbrini E, Klein S. Fundamentals of cardiometabolic risk factor reduction: achieving and maintaining weight loss with pharmacotherapy or bariatric surgery. Clin Cornerstone 2008;9:41–51.
11. Picot J, Jones J, Colquitt JL, et al. The clinical effectiveness and cost-effectiveness of bariatric (weight loss) surgery for obesity: a systematic review and economic evaluation. Health Technol Assess 2009;13:1–190.
12. Dumon KR, Murayama KM. Bariatric surgery outcomes. Surg Clin North Am 2011;91:1313–38.
13. Nguyen NT, Masoomi H, Magno CP, et al. Trends in use of bariatric surgery, 2003–2008. J Am Coll Surg 2011;213:261–6.
14. Sjostrom L, Lindroos AK, Peltonen M. Lifestyle, diabetes, and cardiovascular risk factors 10 years after bariatric surgery. N Engl J Med 2004;351:2683–93.
15. Christou NV, Look D, Maclean LD. Weight gain after short- and long-limb gastric bypass in patients followed for longer than 10 years. Ann Surg 2006;244:734–40.
16. Biron S, Hould FS, Lebel S, et al. Twenty years of biliopancreatic diversion: what is the goal of the surgery? Obes Surg 2004;14:160–4.
17. Reinhold RB. Critical analysis of long term weight loss following gastric bypass. Surg Gynecol Obstet 1982;155:385–94.
18. Magro DO, Geloneze B, Delfini R, et al. Long-term weight regain after gastric bypass: a 5-year prospective study. Obes Surg 2008;18:648–51.
19. Andersen T, Pedersen BH, Dissing I, et al. A randomized comparison of horizontal and vertical banded gastroplasty: what determines weight loss? Scand J Gastroenterol 1989;24:186–92.
20. Salmon PA. Failure of gastroplasty pouch and stoma size to correlate with postoperative weight loss. Can J Surg 1986;29:60–3.
21. Näslund E, Backman L, Granström L, et al. Does the size of the upper pouch affect weight loss after vertical banded gastroplasty? Obes Surg 1995;5:378–81.
22. Kuzmak LI, Burak E. Pouch enlargement: myth or reality? impressions from serial upper gastrointestinal series in silicone gastric banding patients. Obes Surg 1993;3:57–62.

23. Andersen T, Pedersen BH. Pouch volume, stoma diameter, and clinical outcome after gastroplasty for morbid obesity. A prospective study. Scand J Gastroenterol 1984;19:643–9.
24. Flanagan L. Measurement of functional pouch volume following the gastric bypass procedure. Obes Surg 1996;6:38–43.
25. Forsell P. Pouch volume, stoma diameter and weight loss in Swedish adjustable gastric banding (SAGB). Obes Surg 1996;6:468–73.
26. Halverson JD, Koehler RE. Gastric bypass: analysis of weight loss and factors determining success. Surgery 1981;90:446–55.
27. Roberts K, Duffy A, Kaufman J, et al. Size matters: gastric pouch size correlates with weight loss after laparoscopic Roux-en-Y gastric bypass. Surg Endosc 2007; 21:1397–402.
28. Abu Dayyeh BK, Lautz DB, Thompson CC. Gastrojejunal stoma diameter predicts weight regain after Roux-en-Y gastric bypass. Clin Gastroenterol Hepatol 2011;9: 228–33.
29. Heneghan HM, Yimcharoen P, Brethauer SA, et al. Influence of pouch and stoma size on weight loss after gastric bypass. Surg Obes Relat Dis 2012;8(4):408–15.
30. Topart P, Becouarn G, Ritz P. Pouch size after gastric bypass does not correlate with weight loss outcome. Obes Surg 2011;21:1350–4.
31. Hallowell PT, Stellato TA, Yao DA, et al. Should bariatric revisional surgery be avoided secondary to increased morbidity and mortality? Am J Surg 2009;197: 391–6.
32. Zingg U, McQuinn A, DiValentino D, et al. Revisional vs. primary Roux-en-Y gastric bypass–a case-matched analysis: less weight loss in revisions. Obes Surg 2010;20:1627–32.
33. Radtka JF 3rd, Puleo FJ, Wang L, et al. Revisional bariatric surgery: who, what, where, and when? Surg Obes Relat Dis 2010;6:635–42.
34. Morales MP, Wheeler AA, Ramaswamy A, et al. Laparoscopic revisional surgery after Roux-en-Y gastric bypass and sleeve gastrectomy. Surg Obes Relat Dis 2010;6:485–90.
35. Spaulding L. Treatment of dilated gastrojejunostomy with sclerotherapy. Obes Surg 2003;13:254–7.
36. Catalano MF, Rudic G, Anderson AJ, et al. Weight gain after bariatric surgery as a result of a large gastric stoma: endotherapy with sodium morrhuate may prevent the need for surgical revision. Gastrointest Endosc 2007;66:240–5.
37. Spaulding L, Osler T, Patlak J. Long-term results of sclerotherapy for dilated gastrojejunostomy after gastric bypass. Surg Obes Relat Dis 2007;3:623–6.
38. Loewen M, Barba C. Endoscopic sclerotherapy for dilated gastrojejunostomy of failed gastric bypass. Surg Obes Relat Dis 2008;4:539–42.
39. Madan AK, Martinez JM, Khan KA, et al. Endoscopic sclerotherapy for dilated gastrojejunostomy after gastric bypass. J Laparoendosc Adv Surg Tech A 2010;20:235–7.
40. Abu Dayyeh BK, Jirapinyo P, Weitzner Z, et al. Endoscopic sclerotherapy for the treatment of weight regain after Roux-en-Y gastric bypass: outcomes, complications, and predictors of response in 575 procedures. Gastrointest Endosc 2012; 76:275–82.
41. Thompson CC, Slattery J, Bundga ME, et al. Peroral endoscopic reduction of dilated gastrojejunal anastomosis after Roux-en-Y gastric bypass: a possible new option for patients with weight regain. Surg Endosc 2006;20:1744–8.
42. Thompson CC, Roslin MS, Chand B, et al. Restore: randomized evaluation of endoscopic suturing transorally for anastomotic outlet reduction: a double-blind,

sham-controlled multicenter study for treatment of inadequate weight loss or weight regain following Roux-en-Y gastric bypass. Gastroenterology 2010;138:S-388.

43. Mullady DK, Lautz DB, Thompson CC. Treatment of weight regain after gastric bypass surgery when using a new endoscopic platform: initial experience and early outcomes (with video). Gastrointest Endosc 2009;70:440–4.

44. Ryou M, Mullady DK, Lautz DB, et al. Pilot study evaluating technical feasibility and early outcomes of second-generation endosurgical platform for treatment of weight regain after gastric bypass surgery. Surg Obes Relat Dis 2009;5:450–4.

45. Horgan S, Jacobsen G, Weiss GD, et al. Incisionless revision of post-Roux-en-Y bypass stomal and pouch dilation: multicenter registry results. Surg Obes Relat Dis 2010;6:290–5.

46. Thompson CC, Jacobsen GR, Schroder GL, et al. Stoma size critical to 12-month outcomes in endoscopic suturing for gastric bypass repair. Surg Obes Relat Dis 2011;8(3):282–7.

47. Mikami D, Needleman B, Narula V, et al. Natural orifice surgery: initial US experience utilizing the StomaphyX device to reduce gastric pouches after Roux-en-Y gastric bypass. Surg Endosc 2010;24:223–8.

48. Leitman IM, Virk CS, Avgerinos DV, et al. Early results of trans-oral endoscopic plication and revision of the gastric pouch and stoma following Roux-en-Y gastric bypass surgery. JSLS 2010;14:217–20.

49. Manouchehri N, Birch D, Menzes C, et al. Natural orifice surgery: endoluminal pouch reduction following failed vertical banded gastroplasty. Obes Surg 2011; 21:1787–91.

50. Ong'uti SK, Ortega G, Onwugbufor MT, et al. Effective weight loss management with endoscopic gastric plication using StomaphyX device: is it achievable? Surg Obes Relat Dis 2011 Nov 9. [Epub ahead of print].

51. Heylen AM, Jacobs A, Lybeer M, et al. The OTSC(R)-clip in revisional endoscopy against weight gain after bariatric gastric bypass surgery. Obes Surg 2011;21: 1629–33.

52. Benjamin SB. Small bowel obstruction and the Garren-Edwards gastric bubble: an iatrogenic bezoar. Gastrointest Endosc 1988;34:463–7.

53. Benjamin SB, Maher KA, Cattau EL Jr, et al. Double-blind controlled trial of the Garren-Edwards gastric bubble: an adjunctive treatment for exogenous obesity. Gastroenterology 1988;95:581–8.

54. Hogan RB, Johnston JH, Long BW, et al. A double-blind, randomized, sham-controlled trial of the gastric bubble for obesity. Gastrointest Endosc 1989;35: 381–5.

55. Kirby DF, Wade JB, Mills PR, et al. A prospective assessment of the Garren-Edwards gastric bubble and bariatric surgery in the treatment of morbid obesity. Am Surg 1990;56:575–80.

56. Lindor KD, Hughes RW Jr, Ilstrup DM, et al. Intragastric balloons in comparison with standard therapy for obesity–a randomized, double-blind trial. Mayo Clin Proc 1987;62:992–6.

57. Meshkinpour H, Hsu D, Farivar S. Effect of gastric bubble as a weight reduction device: a controlled, crossover study. Gastroenterology 1988;95:589–92.

58. Zeman RK, Benjamin SB, Cunningham MB, et al. Small bowel obstruction due to Garren gastric bubble: radiographic diagnosis. AJR Am J Roentgenol 1988;150: 581–2.

59. Ziessman HA, Collen MJ, Fahey FH, et al. The effect of the Garren-Edwards Gastric Bubble on solid and liquid gastric emptying. Clin Nucl Med 1988;13: 586–9.

60. Geliebter A, Westreich S, Gage D. Gastric distention by balloon and test-meal intake in obese and lean subjects. Am J Clin Nutr 1988;48:592–4.
61. Farina M, Baratta R, Nigro A, et al. Intragastric balloon in association with lifestyle and/or pharmacotherapy in the long-term management of obesity. Obes Surg 2012;22:565–71.
62. Imaz I, Martinez-Cervell C, Garcia-Alvarez EE, et al. Safety and effectiveness of the intragastric balloon for obesity. A meta-analysis. Obes Surg 2008;18:841–6.
63. Papavramidis TS, Grosomanidis V, Papakostas P, et al. Intragastric balloon fundal or antral position affects weight loss and tolerability. Obes Surg 2012;22:904–9.
64. Zerrweck C, Maunoury V, Caiazzo R, et al. Preoperative weight loss with intragastric balloon decreases the risk of significant adverse outcomes of laparoscopic gastric bypass in super-super obese patients. Obes Surg 2012;22:777–82.
65. Genco A, Cipriano M, Bacci V, et al. Intragastric balloon followed by diet vs intragastric balloon followed by another balloon: a prospective study on 100 patients. Obes Surg 2010;20:1496–500.
66. Dumonceau JM, Francois E, Hittelet A, et al. Single vs repeated treatment with the intragastric balloon: a 5-year weight loss study. Obes Surg 2010;20:692–7.
67. Breen DM, Rasmussen BA, Kokorovic A, et al. Jejunal nutrient sensing is required for duodenal-jejunal bypass surgery to rapidly lower glucose concentrations in uncontrolled diabetes. Nat Med 2012;18:950–5.
68. Rodriguez-Grunert L, Galvao Neto MP, Alamo M, et al. First human experience with endoscopically delivered and retrieved duodenal-jejunal bypass sleeve. Surg Obes Relat Dis 2008;4:55–9.
69. Tarnoff M, Rodriguez L, Escalona A, et al. Open label, prospective, randomized controlled trial of an endoscopic duodenal-jejunal bypass sleeve versus low calorie diet for pre-operative weight loss in bariatric surgery. Surg Endosc 2009;23:650–6.
70. Gersin KS, Rothstein RI, Rosenthal RJ, et al. Open-label, sham-controlled trial of an endoscopic duodenojejunal bypass liner for preoperative weight loss in bariatric surgery candidates. Gastrointest Endosc 2010;71:976–82.
71. Rodriguez L, Reyes E, Fagalde P, et al. Pilot clinical study of an endoscopic, removable duodenal-jejunal bypass liner for the treatment of type 2 diabetes. Diabetes Technol Ther 2009;11:725–32.
72. de Moura EG, Martins BC, Lopes GS, et al. Metabolic improvements in obese type 2 diabetes subjects implanted for 1 year with an endoscopically deployed duodenal-jejunal bypass liner. Diabetes Technol Ther 2012;14:183–9.
73. Brethauer SA, Chand B, Schauer PR, et al. Transoral gastric volume reduction as intervention for weight management: 12-month follow-up of TRIM trial. Surg Obes Relat Dis 2012;8:296–303.

Index

Note: Page numbers of article titles are in **boldface** type.

A

Ablation. See specific types, e.g., Thermal ablation
Achalasia, **53–75**
  described, 53
  features of, 53
  management of
    past options, 54
    POEM in, 54–72. See also Peroral endoscopic myotomy (POEM), in achalasia
      management
Adenocarcinoma
  gastric
    prevalence of, 77
Ampullary lesions, **95–109**
  clinical presentation of, 97–98
  described, 96
  diagnosis of, 98–100
  epidemiology of, 96–97
  staging of, 98–100
  treatment of
    alternative techniques in, 105
    endoscopic papillectomy in, 101–104. See also Endoscopic papillectomy,
      in ampullary lesion management
    endoscopic therapy in, 100–101
    surveillance in, 104
APC. See Argon plasma coagulation (APC)
Argon plasma coagulation (APC)
  in early esophageal cancer management, 28
Arteriovenous malformations (AVMs), 115–116
AVMs. See Arteriovenous malformations (AVMs)

B

Balloon strictureplasty
  for small bowel strictures, 116–117
Bariatric leaks and fistulas
  endoscopic therapy for, 126–129
Barrett esophagus
  defined, 1
  described, 1–2
  diagnosis of, 3–4
  endoscopic therapy of, **1–16**

Gastrointest Endoscopy Clin N Am 23 (2013) 177–184
http://dx.doi.org/10.1016/S1052-5157(12)00150-X
1052-5157/13/$ – see front matter © 2013 Elsevier Inc. All rights reserved.

Barrett (*continued*)
      cryotherapy in, 6–7
      endoscopic resection in, 7
      multimodal EET in, 7–10
            candidates for, 8
            complications of, 8–10
      rationale for, 2–3
      RFA in, 5–6
      supporting evidence for, 4–8
   histopathology of, 2–3
   prevalence of, 1–2
   staging of, 3–4
Bleeding
   endoscopic resection of large colon polyps and, 146–147

   C

Cancer(s)
   esophageal
      endoluminal therapy for, **17–39**. See also Esophageal cancer
   gastric
      early, **77–94**. See also Gastric cancer, early
Cholecystectomy
   for pancreaticobiliary leaks and fistulas, 130–131
Colon polyps
   large
      endoscopic resection of, **137–152**
            assessment in, 140–141
            clinical outcomes of, 148–149
            complications of, 146–148
            controversies related to, 149
            follow-up care, 148
            future considerations in, 149
            pedunculated lesions, 141
            postoperative care, 148
            preparation for, 138–140
            reassessment after, 143–145
            sessile and flat lesions, 141–143
            specimen retrieval and preparation in, 145–146
Colonic leaks and fistulas
   endoscopic therapy for, 129–130
Colonic stents
   in malignant bowel obstruction management, 159–161
            bridge to surgery in, 160
            complications of, 161
            indications in, 159–160
            outcomes of, 160
            palliation in, 161
Cryotherapy
   for Barrett esophagus, 6–7
   in early esophageal cancer management, 29

D

Dieulafoy lesions, 119
Distal pancreatectomy
    for pancreaticobiliary leaks and fistulas, 131
DJBL. *See* Duodenal jejunal bypass liner (DJBL)
Duodenal jejunal bypass liner (DJBL)
    in obesity management, 169–170
Dysplasia
    early gastric cancer and, **77–94**

E

EBT. *See* Endoscopic bariatric therapy (EBT)
EET. *See* Endoscopic eradication therapy (EET)
EMR. *See* Endoscopic mucosal resection (EMR)
Endocinch
    for GERD, 46
Endoluminal therapy
    for early gastric cancer
        investigations related to, 84–86
    for esophageal cancer, **17–39**. *See also* Esophageal cancer
    for GERD, **41–51**. *See also* Gastroesophageal reflux disease (GERD), endoluminal
        therapy for
    in small bowel
        general principles of, 112
Endoscopic ablation therapies
    in early esophageal cancer management, 26–29
        APC, 28
        cryotherapy, 29
        PDT, 28–29
        RFA, 26–28
        thermal laser, 28
Endoscopic bariatric therapy (EBT)
    primary
        in obesity management, 168
Endoscopic eradication therapy (EET)
    for Barrett esophagus, 7–10
Endoscopic mucosal resection (EMR)
    in early esophageal cancer management, 21–25
    in early gastric cancer management, 79
Endoscopic papillectomy
    in ampullary lesion management, 101–104
        complications of, 104
        electrocautery settings in, 103
        en bloc or piecemeal resection in, 101–103
        endoscopic resection in, 101
        postresection sphincterotomy in, 104
        preresection sphincterotomy in, 103–104
        submucosal injection in, 101
        thermal ablation in, 103
        tissue retrieval and postprocedure inspection in, 103

Endoscopic resection
  in ampullary lesion management, 101
  in early esophageal cancer management, 21–26
      EDS, 25–26
      EMR, 21–25
  in early gastric cancer management, 79–83
  of large colon polyps, **137–152**. See also Colon polyps, large, endoscopic resection of
Endoscopic retrograde cholangiopancreatography (ERCP)
  in ampullary lesion diagnosis, 99–100
Endoscopic submucosal dissection (ESD)
  in early esophageal cancer management, 25–26
  in early gastric cancer management, 80–83
Endoscopic therapy. See specific types and indications
Endoscopic ultrasound (EUS)
  in ampullary lesion diagnosis, 98–99
  in early gastric cancer evaluation, 78–79
Endoscopy
  in ampullary lesion diagnosis, 98
  in obesity management, **165–175**. See also Obesity, management of, endoscopy in
Enteral stents
  for small bowel strictures, 117–118
ERCP. See Endoscopic retrograde cholangiopancreatography (ERCP)
ESD. See Endoscopic submucosal dissection (ESD)
Esophageal cancer
  early
      management of, 18–29
          endoscopic ablation therapies in, 26–29
          endoscopic resection in, 21–26. See also Endoscopic resection, in early
              esophageal cancer management
          operative resection in, 18–19
          staging in, 19–21
      endoluminal therapy for, **17–39**
      features of, 18
      palliation of, 30–33
      prevalence of, 17
      SEMSs in, 30–33
Esophageal leaks and fistulas
  endoscopic therapy for, 124–126
EUS. See Endoscopic ultrasound (EUS)

  F

Familial adenomatous polyposis (FAP) syndrome, 114
FAP syndrome. See Familial adenomatous polyposis (FAP) syndrome
Fistula(s)
  postoperative
      endoscopic therapy for, **123–136**. See also specific types

  G

Gastric adenocarcinoma
  prevalence of, 77

Gastric cancer
    early, **77–94**
        dysplasia and, **77–94**
        evaluation of
            EUS in, 78–79
            pretreatment, 78
        treatment of, 79–86
            considerations in, 78
            endoluminal therapy in
                investigations related to, 84–86
            endoscopic resection in, 79–83
            future directions in, 86–87
            Helicobacter pylori infection–related, 83–84
            molecular techniques in, 87
            ongoing clinical investigations in, 86
            robotic surgery in, 87
            surgical resection in, 83
            surveillance for metachronous gastric cancer in, 83
    metachronous
        surveillance for
            in early gastric cancer management, 83
Gastroduodenal stents
    in malignant bowel obstruction management,
        156–159
        complications of, 159
        indications for, 156–158
        outcomes of, 158–159
Gastroesophageal reflux disease (GERD)
    described, 41–42
    endoluminal therapy for, **41–51**
        complications of, 48–49
        Endocinch, 46
        follow-up after, 46
        future directions in, 49
        indications for, 42–43
        procedural techniques, 43–46
            TIF, 43–44
        results of, 47–48
        Stretta procedure, 44–46
GERD. *See* Gastroesophageal reflux disease (GERD)

H

Helicobacter pylori infection
    treatment of
        in early gastric cancer management,
            83–84
Hepatic resection
    for pancreaticobiliary leaks and fistulas, 131
Hepatic transplant
    for pancreaticobiliary leaks and fistulas, 131

I

Intragastric balloon
    in obesity management, 168–169

L

Laser therapy
    thermal laser
        in early esophageal cancer management, 28
Leak(s)
    postoperative
        endoscopic therapy for, **123–136**. *See also specific types*
Lesion(s)
    ampullary, **95–109**. *See also* Ampullary lesions
    in small intestine, **111–121**. *See also specific types*

M

Malignant bowel obstruction
    SEMSs in, **153–164**. *See also* Self-expanding metal stents (SEMSs), in malignant bowel
        obstruction management
Molecular techniques
    in early gastric cancer management, 87

N

Nonampullary duodenal polyps, 114–115

O

Obesity
    management of
        described, 165–166
        endoscopy in, **165–175**
            described, 166–167
            DJBL, 169–170
            intragastric balloon, 168–169
            primary EBT, 168
            transoral gastic volume reduction, 170–171

P

Pancreatectomy
    distal
        for pancreaticobiliary leaks and fistulas, 131
Pancreaticobiliary leaks and fistulas
    endoscopic therapy for, 130–131
PDT. *See* Photodynamic therapy (PDT)
Perforation
    endoscopic resection of large colon polyps and, 147–148
Peroral endoscopic myotomy (POEM)
    in achalasia management, 54–72
        complications of, 65

contraindications to, 56–57
controversies related to, 67–70
equipment in, 57–60
future considerations in, 70–72
indications for, 56–57
outcomes of, 65–67
patient preparation for, 57
postoperative care, 65
technique, 60–64
described, 54–55
Peutz-Jeghers syndrome (PJS), 112–114
Photodynamic therapy (PDT)
in early esophageal cancer management, 28–29
PJS. *See* Peutz-Jeghers syndrome (PJS)
POEM. *See* Peroral endoscopic myotomy (POEM)
Polyp(s)
colon
large
endoscopic resection of, **137–152**. *See also* Colon polyps, large, endoscopic
resection of
small bowel, 112–115
Preresection sphincterotomy
in ampullary lesion management, 103–104
Primary endoscopic bariatric therapy
in obesity management, 168

R

Radiofrequency ablation (RFA)
for Barrett esophagus, 5–6
in early esophageal cancer management, 26–28
RFA. *See* Radiofrequency ablation (RFA)
Robotic surgery
in early gastric cancer management, 87

S

Self-expanding metal stents (SEMSs)
in early esophageal cancer management, 30–33
in malignant bowel obstruction management, **153–164**
colonic stents, 159–161
gastroduodenal stents, 156–159
techniques, 155–156
technology related to, 153–154
SEMSs. *See* Self-expanding metal stents (SEMSs)
Small bowel polyps, 112–115
Small bowel strictures, 116–118
Small bowel tumors, 119
Small intestine
endoluminal therapy in
general principles of, 112
lesions in, **111–121**. *See also specific types*

Sphincterotomy
  postresection
    in ampullary lesion management, 104
  preresection
    in ampullary lesion management, 103–104
Stent(s). *See also specific types*
  colonic
    in malignant bowel obstruction management, 159–161
  enteral
    for small bowel strictures, 117–118
  gastroduodenal
    in malignant bowel obstruction management, 156–159
Stretta procedure
  for GERD, 44–46
Stricture(s)
  small bowel, 116–118
Strictureplasty
  balloon
    for small bowel strictures, 116–117
Submucosal injection
  in ampullary lesion management, 101
Surgical resection
  in early gastric cancer management, 83

T

Thermal ablation
  in ampullary lesion management, 103
Thermal laser
  in early esophageal cancer management, 28
TIF. *See* Transoral incisionless fundoplication (TIF)
Transoral gastric volume reduction
  in obesity management, 170–171
Transoral incisionless fundoplication (TIF)
  for GERD, 43–44
Transplantation
  hepatic
    for pancreaticobiliary leaks and fistulas, 131
Tumor(s)
  small bowel, 119

U

Ultrasound
  endoscopic. *See* Endoscopic ultrasound (EUS)

Moving?

Make sure your subscription moves with you!

To notify us of your new address, find your **Clinics Account Number** (located on your mailing label above your name), and contact customer service at:

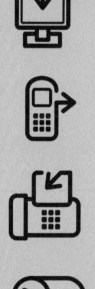

Email: journalscustomerservice-usa@elsevier.com

800-654-2452 (subscribers in the U.S. & Canada)
314-447-8871 (subscribers outside of the U.S. & Canada)

Fax number: 314-447-8029

Elsevier Health Sciences Division
Subscription Customer Service
3251 Riverport Lane
Maryland Heights, MO 63043

*To ensure uninterrupted delivery of your subscription, please notify us at least 4 weeks in advance of move.

Printed and bound by CPI Group (UK) Ltd, Croydon, CR0 4YY

03/10/2024

01040431-0012